New Hope for Mental Disturbances

NEW HOPE FOR MENTAL DISTURBANCES

VLADIMIR LERNER
AND
CHANOCH MIODOWNIK
EDITORS

Nova Science Publishers, Inc.
New York

For permission to use material from this book please contact us:
Telephone 631-231-7269; Fax 631-231-8175
Web Site: http://www.novapublishers.com

LIBRARY OF CONGRESS CATALOGING-IN-PUBLICATION DATA

New hope for mental disturbances / [edited by] Vladimir Lerner and Chanoch Miodownik.
p. cm.
Includes index.
ISBN 978-1-60692-691-8 (hardcover)
1. Mental illness--Treatment. 2. Vitamin therapy. 3. Vitamins. I. Lerner, Vladimir. II. Miodownik, Chanoch.
RC454.4.N493 2009
616.89'18--dc22

2008053065

Published by Nova Science Publishers, Inc. ✢ New York

CONTENTS

PREFACE

The purpose of this book is to introduce the importance of vitamins and its use in the treatment of schizophrenia, mood and movement disorders. This subject has been already known for many years. In the last years this issue has become "hot" again. To date there is new modern data based on controlled studies leading to a new attitude in consumption of these preparations. The present experience is related to higher doses in contrast to those which were used previously in addition to the scientific base data consisting of new knowledge about the mechanism of action and the influence on different dimensions. The chapters will include theoretical and scientific background as well as practical data based conclusions which might be useful for the clinician in everyday practice.

Introduction - The Tsadik eats to satisfy his soul" (Proverbs 13:25)

"Excessive intake of food is like poison to the human body and is the root cause of many illnesses. Most of the illnesses that strike people are caused either by bad foods or because people fill their stomachs with too much food, even when the foods are good. As King Solomon said in his wisdom: "One who guards his mouth and tongue keeps his soul from troubles" (Proverbs 21:23) - in other words, when he guards his mouth from eating bad foods or from overeating, and his tongue from speaking unnecessarily.") Maimonides, Hilchot Deot 4:15

"The main work of the doctors should be in the area of food and drink: to warn people what to avoid, and to give instructions about what to eat." (Ramban on Leviticus 26:11)

Let food be your medicine (Hippocrates 460BC)

Chapter 1 - Vitamin C is a *water-soluble nutrient* and human *vitamin* essential for life and for maintaining optimal health, used by the body for many purposes. It is also known by the chemical name of its principal form, L-ascorbic acid. Ascorbic acid can be broken down by ascorbic acid oxidase an enzyme which catalyses the oxidation of ascorbic acid.

Almost all animals and plants synthesize their own vitamin C. There are some exceptions, such as *humans* and a small number of other animals, including, *apes, guinea pigs,* the *red-vented bulbul*, a fruit-eating bat and species of trout.

Vitamin C was first isolated in 1928, and in 1932 it was proved to be the agent that prevents scurvy, however, from the 1930s, some practitioners experimented with vitamin C as a treatment for diseases other than scurvy.

In the brain, the nerve endings contain the highest concentrations of vitamin C in the human body (after the suprarenal glands). Vitamin C is important and necessary for the synthesis of the neurotransmitters: norepinephrine and serotonin. It catalyzes the conversion of dopamine to norepinephrine and the conversion of tryptophan to serotonin.

We obtained all available information in medical literature and internet resources about vitamin C using, concerning its relations to psychiatric disturbances.

This chapter describes vitamin C biological functions, discovery and the debate on how it is used by society. Moreover, we summarize data regarding use of vitamin C in psychiatric practice in particularly in schizophrenia, mood in related disorders, Alzheimer's disease, attention deficit hyperactivity disorder, and others.

Chapter 2 - Vitamin B_6 gained immense significance with the discovery in the 1940s of its important role in animal and human nutrition. It is involved in about 100 enzymatic reactions in the body. The most important of these are transamination, decarboxylation, cleavage reactions, substance synthesis, transsulfhydration, desulfhydration, and racemization. Vitamin B_6 deficiency causes a broad spectrum of both physical and mental symptoms. The aims of this chapter were to summarize contemporary data concerning 1) vitamin B_6 and psychotic symptoms; 2) its influence on homocysteine serum level; and 3) vitamin B_6 use for psychotropic drug-induced movement disorders. The data cumulated to date demonstrate that vitamin B_6 may be effective in treating psychotropic drug-induced movement disorders, as in the case of acute movement disturbances as well as tardive movement disorders. The influence on psychotic symptoms was not confirmed, and further studies with higher doses of the vitamin are indicated.

"Megavitamin treatment does not work magically, overnight, like drugs." —*Dr. Abram Hoffer*

Chapter 3 - Depression is one of the frequent and disabling conditions in the world. About 10% of the population suffers from a kind of clinical depression. Sometimes it is difficult to differ whether it is a primary problem, but during the last decades more have been known about the combinations of depressive states and deficiency of at least one nutrient. Mood disorders are associated with heterogeneous dysregulation of the biogenic amines. Norepinephrine and serotonin have an important role in etiology of depression. The cholinergic, dopaminergic, and GABA system have also been associated with depression.

One of the possible explanations for the aetiology of depression, related to serotonin theory, is that vitamin B6 which is a key enzyme involved in the synthesis of different neurotransmitters and its deficiency may lead to appearance of depression.

Depression is not a crime. But it plummets a person into an abyss deeper than any crime could reach. Rabbi Menachem M. Schneerson [1]

Chapter 4 - The initial clinical importance of folate and vitamin B12 (cobalamin) was related to their role in the development of macrocytic anemia. However, it subsequently became clear that these essential dietary substances played an important role in the functioning of the nervous system. Today there is increasing evidence that hematological and neuropsychiatric effects due to cobalamin and folate deficiency do not necessarily occur simultaneously. Mental or psychological changes may precede hematological signs by months or years, and they may in fact represent the initial or only symptoms.

The relationship between cobalamin and folate deficiency and psychiatric illness has been studied since these vitamins were first discovered in the 1940's. The mental effects described in the context of cobalamin deficiency cover a wide range of symptoms, varying from cognitive impairment (slow mentation, memory deficits, confusion, dementia), to mood changes (agitation, depression, mania) and even to psychotic episodes (paranoia, auditory and visual hallucinations, delusions). There is a clear association between folate and cognitive and mood disorders.

Chapter 5 - Homocysteine (Hcy) is an amino acid generated via methionine metabolism suggested to be rapidly taken up by neurons via a specific membrane transporter. Several enzymes, including methylenetetrahydrofolate reductase, methionine synthase and cystathionine beta-synthase, are involved in homocysteine metabolism and vitamins B_{12} and B_6 and folate serve as co-factors for these and other enzymes involved in homocysteine metabolism.

Homocysteine is suggested to be a neurotoxic amino acid via its effects on the NMDA receptors and/or the cell redox status.

Elevated plasma homocysteine has been found to be a risk factor for Alzheimer's disease as well as cerebral vascular disease, suggesting that some risk factors can accelerate or increase the severity of several CNS disease processes.

We screened 193 chronic schizophrenic patients from our region for plasma homocysteine levels and compared them with 762 controls (evaluated in a screening program for employee health). Mean homocysteine level was 16.3 ± 11.8 (SD) μM in schizophrenic patients vs. 10.6 ± 3.6 (SD) μM in healthy controls. The elevation in homocysteine was statistically significant and was evident almost entirely in young male schizophrenic patients. A second study in 184 consecutively admitted schizophrenic patients and 305 control subjects showed similar results.

Homocysteine can be lowered by providing oral folic acid, vitamin B_{12} and pyridoxine. Forty-two schizophrenic patients with plasma homocysteine levels above 15 μM were treated either with these vitamins for three months or placebo for three months in a randomized double-blind placebo controlled crossover design. Homocysteine levels significantly declined on vitamin therapy compared to placebo in all patients except for one non-compliant subject. Clinical symptoms of schizophrenia as measured by the Positive and Negative Syndrome Scale (PANSS) declined significantly more in those on active treatment compared with placebo. Of the neuropsychological test results, the Wisconsin Card Sort (Categories Completed) results were significantly better after vitamin treatment than after placebo.

A subgroup of schizophrenic patients with hyperhomocysteinemia may thus benefit from the addition of B vitamins, a fairly simple therapeutic strategy.

Chapter 6 - Omega-3 fatty acids are considered essential fatty acids. They are essential to human health, but cannot be manufactured by the body. In recent years, researchers have demonstrated a growing interest in fatty acids and their beneficial influence on human health. Positive findings have multiplied, and more than 500 papers on this topic have been published during the last 70 years. Omega-3 fatty acids are built in to the cell membrane, affecting the function of neurotransmitter receptors. A relationship appears to exist between omega-3 fatty acids and central nervous system (CNS) neurotransmitters. It has been shown that oil diets may have mood-stabilizing effects by reducing the generation of second messengers coming from phosphatidylinositol and phosphatidylcholine in cell membranes. It was suggested that major depression is associated with elevated plasma concentrations of the 2-series prostaglandins (PGE2). Other suggested actions of omega-3 fatty acids include reduction in proinflammatory cytokines, direct inhibition of PKC activity and alteration in serotonergic neurotransmission. Omega-3 fatty acids are believed to stimulate neurotrophic factor, increasing synaptic plasticity, improving neurotransmission, and to have antidepressant and neuroprotective properties.

Chapter 7 - Although antipsychotic drugs are an indispensable component of the management of schizophrenia, clinical response of psychopathological symptoms, cognitive impairment, quality of life and elevated emotional distress remains incomplete in schizophrenia. Consequently the development of more effective treatments is an important research goal. One promising direction is the use of neuroprotective agents. This review will focus on the evidence from clinical and basic science studies supporting a role of several potential neuroprotective compounds, representing a wide range of mechanisms, such as neurosteroids (pregnenolone, dehydroepiandrosterone), memantine, bexarotene and L-theanine. Neuroprotective effects of these agents as add-on therapies merit further investigation in schizophrenia and related disorders.

Chapter 8 - In recent years the spectrum of known effects of melatonin was reported to exceed by far the original discoveries. Melatonin regulates, circadian and seasonal rhythms, such as the sleep-wake cycle and acts as an immunostimulator and cytoprotective agent. The association between melatonin and schizophrenia has been studied in several clinical domains such as sleep, cognition and tardive dyskinesia. The presumed pathophysiology and mechanism is thought to be related to the regulation of central dopaminergic pathways. In addition, recent clinical and research data indicates that melatonin may be advantageous as a complementary intervention for sleep disturbances of schizophrenia patients and possibly for patients suffering from tardive dyskinesia.

In: New Hope for Mental Disturbances
Editors: Vladimir Lerner and Chanoch Meodownik
ISBN 978-1-60692-691-8

INTRODUCTION: FOOD SUPPLEMENTS – A NEW HOPE FOR SCHIZOPHRENIA AND MOOD DISORDERS

Vladimir Lerner[1] and Chanoch Miodownik
Mental Health Center, Faculty of Health Sciences Ben-Gurion University of the Negev, Be'er-Sheva, Israel

INTRODUCTION

Vitamins (and Food Supplements) and its Role in Nature (Mental Health)

The Tsadik eats to satisfy his soul" (Proverbs 13:25)

"Excessive intake of food is like poison to the human body and is the root cause of many illnesses. Most of the illnesses that strike people are caused either by bad foods or because people fill their stomachs with too much food, even when the foods are good. As King Solomon said in his wisdom: "One who guards his mouth and tongue keeps his soul from troubles" (Proverbs 21:23) - in other words, when he guards his mouth from eating bad foods or from overeating, and his tongue from speaking unnecessarily.") Maimonides, Hilchot Deot 4:15

"The main work of the doctors should be in the area of food and drink: to warn people what to avoid, and to give instructions about what to eat." (Ramban on Leviticus 26:11)

Let food be your medicine (Hippocrates 460BC)

The relations between mental, spiritual states and nutrition are known for thousands of years. As we can see in the examples above many ancient philosophers and physicians have dealt with this theme. This subject was neglected in the modern medicine, but among natural therapists (naturopaths) the use of food supplements and natural components (health food)

1 Corresponding author: Vladimir Lerner, Faculty of Health Sciences, Ben Gurion University of the Negev and Director of the Psychiatric Department at Be'er Sheva Mental Health Center. Mail address: Be'er Sheva Mental Health Center, PO Box 4600, Be'er Sheva 84170, Israel, Tel.: +972 8 6401408; Fax: +972 8 6401491; Email: lernervld@yahoo.com.

continued to be very popular. The popularity of health food for a long time was based, generally, on clinical daily life impression without any scientific database.

The word vitamine was coined at the Lister Institute in London by the Polish biochemist Kazimierz Funk commonly anglicized as Casimir Funk (1884-1967) in 1912. He was generally credited with the first formulation of the concept of Vitamins, which he called vital amines or vitamines. Vita in Latin is life and the - amine suffix is for amine; at the time it was thought that all vitamins were amines. In 1920, British biochemist Sir Jack Cecil Drummond (1891-1952) proposed that the final "e" be dropped, to deemphasize the "amine" reference, after the discovery that vitamin C had no amine component, and the name has been "vitamin" ever since.

The reason the alphabet soup of vitamins seems to skip from E to the rarely-mentioned K is that most of the "letters" were reclassified, as with fatty acids, discarded as false leads, or renamed because of their relationship to "vitamin B", which became a "complex" of vitamins. Vitamin G, Riboflavin, for example, is now known as B_2. Throughout the early 1900s, scientists were able to isolate and identify a number of vitamins by depriving animals of them. Initially, lipid from fish oil was used to cure rickets in rats, and the fat-soluble nutrient was called "antirachitic A". The irony here is that the first "vitamin" bioactivity ever isolated, which cured rickets, was initially called vitamin A, this bioactivity is now called vitamin D, which is itself subject to the semantic debate that it is not truly a vitamin because it is a steroid derivative. What we now call "vitamin A" was identified in fish oil because it was inactivated by ultraviolet light. Most of what we now recognize as the water-soluble organic micronutrients were initially referred to as just one entity, "vitamin B".

Many trivial health behaviors were not always so conventional. It was slowly developed and some times it was a matter of co-incidence or anecdotal event. There are many examples for that, some of them will be introduced below.

The value of eating certain foods to maintain health was recognized long before vitamins were identified. The ancient Egyptians knew that feeding a patient liver, would help to cure night blindness, now known to be caused by a vitamin A deficiency.

Many “mysterious” illnesses were described and finally found to be connected to specific nutritional elements. Interesting example is beriberi which is caused by thiamin deficiency. Although the disease was described by the ancient Chinese (2697 BC), the relationship with thiamin deficiency was recognized by chance only in 1937. The beriberi syndrome consisted of a series of symptoms that were particularly noxious in samurai Japan: sheepishness, that is, inattention or stupor (not a desired quality in samurai), outbursts of anger (themselves potentially fatal if directed to a member of a higher class), lethargy, loss of appetite, tingling in the fingers and toes, labored breathing, quickened pulse, and, finally, death. Healthy soldiers in fighting form could fall ill and die in as little as two hours. Death usually occurred two hours after the midday meal, and it was gruesome. Unfortunately, nations, like people, forget the lessons learned in history, including the lessons of the history of vitamins. By 1860, Japan was once again faced with a beriberi crisis.

In 1878 alone, the Dutch lost 690 native laborers, and the Dutch colonial health officer on Sumatra recorded, "On average, transport by ship to Java...has taken ten lives per ship." In 1879 so many had died of beriberi there was a shortage of gravediggers to bury them. The government in The Hague sent a young bacteriologist, Christiaan Eijkman (1858 -1830) future the Nobel Prize in Physiology or Medicine 1929, to solve the problem. For eleven years he did the things bacteriologist do, trying to find the germ that caused the disease.

White rice was considered a better food than brown rice in Eijkman's time, and brown rice was usually fed to the chickens. Recently, however, Dr. Eijkman's servants had had too much white rice and fed it to the poultry. Dr. Eijkman quickly concluded he had seen the first-ever case of beriberi in chickens. The cure for beriberi, Dr. Eijkman was sure, was as simple as finding what the poison was in white rice. Not aware that he was writing the first chapter in the history of vitamins, for the next five years Eijkman experimented with every conceivable variation of rice as chicken feed.

He served the chicken rice in stone pots. Then he tried wooden pots, metal pots, and coconut shells. He boiled the rice in well water, in stream water, and in distilled water. He gave the chickens white rice, brown rice, red rice, blue rice, and black rice, husked rice and unhusked rice, and every possible combination thereof.

It wasn't an amazing discovery to the scientists of the day because they didn't get a chance to read about it. Dr. Eijkman published his results in a paper in Dutch read all across Dutch Batavia, by perhaps a dozen persons, and was allowed to go home.

Another interesting issue is why is it so important to eat citrus fruits? It was not known until 1747, when the Scottish surgeon James Lind (1716-1794) discovered that citrus foods helped to prevent scurvy, a particularly deadly disease in which collagen is not properly formed, and characterized by poor wound healing, bleeding of the gums, and severe pain. In 1753, Lind published his Treatise on the Scurvy. His recommendation of using lemons and limes to avoid scurvy was adopted by the British Royal Navy. His discovery, however, was not widely accepted by individuals. In the Royal Navy's Arctic expeditions in the 19th century, for example, it was widely believed that scurvy was prevented by good hygiene on board ship, regular exercise, and maintaining the morale of the crew, rather than by a diet of fresh food, so that Navy expeditions took all the amenities of 'sophisticated' society, like silk sheets, spices, expensive food and drink, and almost nothing of any use beyond the Arctic Circle. As a result, these expeditions continued to be plagued by scurvy and other deficiency diseases. At the time Robert Falcon Scott (1868-1912) made his two expeditions to the Antarctic in the early 20th century, the prevailing medical theory was that scurvy was caused by "tainted" canned food.

Every modern woman might know the advantages of breast feeding. Once the natural mother milk contains many essential components, it has a highly important role in development of babies. These facts were not so familiar until the end of the 19th century.

In 1881, Russian surgeon Nikolai Lunin (1853-1937) fed mice upon an artificial mixture of all the separate constituents of milk known at that time, namely the proteins, fats, carbohydrates, and salts. They died, while the mice fed by milk itself developed normally. He made a conclusion that "a natural food such as milk must therefore contain besides these known principal ingredients small quantities of unknown substances essential to life". However, his conclusion was rejected by other researchers who were unable to reproduce his results. One difference was that he used table sugar (sucrose), while other researchers used milk sugar (lactose) which still contained small amounts of vitamin B.

Scientists now have shifted their focus to discovering ways, in which vitamins can promote health, prevent disease, boost the body's protection against infection and even slow down the aging process. At the same time, public interest in vitamins has heightened. This has been prompted by headlines in the media and widespread advertising by the manufacturers of nutrient supplements.

Each vitamin has specific functions. If levels of a particular vitamin are inadequate, a result is deficiency disease. Deficiencies of vitamins are either primary or secondary. A primary deficiency occurs because there are no enough vitamins in the consumpted food. A secondary deficiency may be due to a lifestyle factor, such as smoking, excessive alcohol consumption, or the use of certain medications that interfere with the absorption or the body's use of the vitamin.

There are few classic examples as mentioned above, but it should be noted that there are some vitamin deficiencies induced by another pathology. In these cases the vitamin deficiency is a by product of conditions like intrinsic factor deficiency in the small bowel or special intestinal bacterial flora, which cause vitamin B_{12} deficiency. Excessive alcohol consumption may lead in extreme cases to Korsakoff's syndrome in which people suffered from vitamin $B_{1,}$ also called thiamine deficiency. This is a very important example concerning mental health and nutrition, because the patient develops amnestic disorder. The syndrome is characterized by a severe memory defect, especially for recent event, for which the patient compensates by confabulation - inventing events to fill the gaps in memory.

One of the main reasons that alcoholism leads to thiamine deficiency has to do with the high-calorie nature of alcohol. A person with a large alcohol intake often, in essence, substitutes alcohol for other, more nutritive calorie sources. Food intake drops off considerably, and multiple vitamin deficiencies develop. Furthermore, it is believed that alcohol increases the body's requirements for B vitamins, at the same time interfering with the absorption of thiamine from the intestine and impairing the body's ability to store and use thiamine. Direct neurotoxic (poisonous damage to the nerves) effects of alcohol may also play some role.

Other nutritional deficiencies often first appear in the form of mental symptoms. For example, depression may be caused by an amino acid imbalance or vitamin deficiency. The B-Vitamins, folic acid, and omega-3 fatty acid may be helpful for regulating stress and balancing mood. St. John's Wort and Kava Kava may help with depression and anxiety.

The past few decades have seen a major advance in the understanding of mental illnesses. It is now clearly understood that schizophrenia, bipolar depression, and other mental disorders are primarily caused by imbalances in brain neurotransmitters. Stressful events and flawed life experiences are now viewed as aggravating factors that may trigger a breakdown in mental functioning, but not a primary cause. The modern psychiatry has found new agents to relieve mental symptoms, but it is already clear that there are limitations which we have to face with. The new horizon of vitamins and other natural supplements can be useful as augmentation agents and relief of the patient's agony. The last decade development of psychiatric researches protruded the scientific proofs for these agents' efficacy. There are many professional medical publications in appreciated journals dealing with such studies.

This book will summarize the current body of knowledge about importance of vitamins and food supplements on the main mental illnesses from an advanced modern point of view.

In: New Hope for Mental Disturbances
Editors: Vladimir Lerner and Chanoch Meodownik
ISBN 978-1-60692-691-8

Chapter 1

VITAMIN C IN PSYCHIATRY: PAST, PRESENT AND FUTURE

Joseph Bergman and Anatoly Kreinin [1]
Mental Health Center Tirat Carmel,
Technion – Rappaport Faculty of Medicine, Haifa, Israel

ABSTRACT

Vitamin C is a *water-soluble nutrient* and human *vitamin* essential for life and for maintaining optimal health, used by the body for many purposes. It is also known by the chemical name of its principal form, L-ascorbic acid. Ascorbic acid can be broken down by ascorbic acid oxidase an enzyme which catalyses the oxidation of ascorbic acid.

Almost all animals and plants synthesize their own vitamin C. There are some exceptions, such as *humans* and a small number of other animals, including, *apes, guinea pigs,* the *red-vented bulbul*, a fruit-eating bat and species of trout.

Vitamin C was first isolated in 1928, and in 1932 it was proved to be the agent that prevents scurvy, however, from the 1930s, some practitioners experimented with vitamin C as a treatment for diseases other than scurvy.

In the brain, the nerve endings contain the highest concentrations of vitamin C in the human body (after the suprarenal glands). Vitamin C is important and necessary for the synthesis of the neurotransmitters: norepinephrine and serotonin. It catalyzes the conversion of dopamine to norepinephrine and the conversion of tryptophan to serotonin.

We obtained all available information in medical literature and internet resources about vitamin C using, concerning its relations to psychiatric disturbances.

This chapter describes vitamin C biological functions, discovery and the debate on how it is used by society. Moreover, we summarize data regarding use of vitamin C in psychiatric practice in particularly in schizophrenia, mood in related disorders, Alzheimer's disease, attention deficit hyperactivity disorder, and others.

---

1 Corresponding author: Anatoly Kreinin, Technion – Rappaport Faculty of Medicine, Department at the Tirat Carmel Mental Health Center. Mail address: Mental Health Center Tirat Carmel, str. Eyala, 17, Tirat Carmel, 30200, PO Box 9, Israel, Tel.: +972 4 8559325; Fax: +97248559325; Email: kranat@netvision.net.il.

History of Vitamin C

Having the right molecules in the right amounts in the right place in the human body at the right time is a necessary condition for good health.

Linus Pauling

The need to include fresh plant food or raw animal flesh in the diet to prevent disease was known from ancient times. Native peoples living in marginal areas incorporated this into their medicinal lore. For example, infusions of spruce needles were used in the temperate zones, or the leaves from species of drought-resistant trees in desert areas. The British navy did not adopt lemon or lime juice until 1795 as standard issue at sea. In the seventeenth century a ships surgeon to the East India Company, one Richard Woodall recommended the use of lemon juice as a preventive and cure in his book ‘Surgeon's Mate’. The first attempt to give scientific basis for the cause of scurvy was by a ships surgeon in the British Royal Navy, James Lind (1716 - 1794). His test was conducted at sea in May 1747 and consisted of two groups of men. One group was provided with lemon juice in addition to their normal rations, the other was not. This test was considered to be the first example of a controlled experiment comparing results on two populations of a factor applied to one group only with all other factors the same. The results of the tests conclusively showed that lemons prevented the disease. Lind published it in 1753.

Vitamin C, or ascorbic acid, is water-soluble and easily destroyed. Unlike most mammals, humans do not have the ability to make their own vitamin C. Therefore, people must obtain vitamin C through their diet. It is essential in wound healing and in the formation of collagen, a protein important in the formation of healthy skin, tendons, bones, and supportive tissues. Vitamin C is also known as, L-ascorbic acid, dehydroascorbic acid, the antiscorbutic vitamin, L-xyloascorbic acid and L-threo-hex-2-uronic acidy-lactone, is a much talked about vitamin, with people claiming it as a cure-all for may diseases and problems - from cancer to the common cold.

To put this saga in proper perspective, we should begin this tale about 60 million years ago. For that is when, according to biochemist Dr. Irwin Stone, our ancestors lost the ability to make their own vitamin C [1-6]. But we did not lose our requirement for considerable amounts of this life-sustaining and critical nutrient on a daily basis. Our loss of self-sufficiency with respect to vitamin C and our subsequent dependence upon diet to provide adequate amounts has impacted significantly our health and lifestyle throughout history, relevant especially today in our polluted, nutrient-depleted, stressful high-tech "advanced" world. We have indeed traveled (fallen) a long way since our proverbial exit from the paradisiacal garden of Eden, where presumably there was an abundance of citrus fruits and vitamin C.

Time warp - Middle Ages. Sailors expiring by droves – exhaustion, depression, muscle pain, haggard appearance, bleeding gums, stinking breath, hemorrhaging and extensive bruising, diarrhea, lung/kidney troubles and death. Scurvy. Dead sailors of all nationalities – Portuguese, Spanish, British, French. Horrible voyages, many corpses and countless unaccomplished missions.

1536. The French explorer Jacques Cartier (1491-1557), exploring the St. Lawrence River, used the local natives' knowledge to save his men who were dying of scurvy. He boiled the needles of the arbor vitae tree to make a tea that was later shown to contain 50 mg of vitamin C per 100 grams. Iroquois Indian remedy for scurvy – tea made from the leaves and bark of the arbor vitae tree determined, centuries later, to possess high vitamin C content.

1747. Another experiment consisted of two groups of men. One group was provided with lemon juice in addition to their normal rations, the other was not. This test was considered to be the first example of a controlled experiment comparing results on two populations of a factor applied to one group only with all other factors the same. The results of the tests conclusively showed that lemons prevented the disease. Lind published it in 1753. The British navy did not adopt lemon or lime juice until 1795 as standard issue at sea. In today's world obsessed with double-blind placebo-controlled trials, Lind's work would have been criticized on the basis of the small sample size, lack of placebo and lack of double blind. The British Admiralty, despite the huge losses incurred from this devastating condition, waited 48 years until 1795 before decreeing that daily rations of fresh lime juice be given to sailors in the British Navy. Although scurvy disappeared very soon thereafter from the British Navy, it continued its scourge throughout the British merchant marine for another 70 years, until the Board of Trade followed suit with a similar decree in 1865.

1911. Theory of "vitamins" published by Polish biochemist Casimir Funk (1884-1967) working in London, theorizing that four substances found in natural foods confer protection against the diseases of beriberi, rickets, pellagra and scurvy. In 1913 the American E.V. McCollum (1879-1967) started the modern nomenclature system of vitamins, by referring to "fat-soluble A", "water-soluble B", scurvy-preventing "water-soluble C" and rickets-preventing "fat-soluble D".

1928. First isolation of pure vitamin C by Hungarian biochemist Albert Szent-Györgyi (1893–1986) working in Cambridge England, the Mayo Clinic, Minnesota and Hungary [2-6]. Szent-Györgyi isolated a substance which he named hexuronic acid, and which was subsequently shown, in 1932, to be vitamin C by American scientists W.A. Waugh and Charles Glen King (1896-1988) [3]. Typical of so many scientific discoveries, Szent-Györgyi was not actually searching for vitamin C. He was attempting to identify an oxygen-combining substance which prevents the appearance of brown pigment from decaying fruit. His diverse expertises in oxidation-reaction and physiology enabled him to isolate a large enough quantity of hexuronic acid from cabbages, adrenal glands of animals, as well as that favorite Hungarian spice, paprika. Following the determination by Szent-Györgyi of the substance's chemical formula $C_6H_8O_6$, and the determination of its structural formula in collaboration with the English chemist Haworth, the chemical name for vitamin C was changed from hexuronic to ascorbic acid, denoting an acidic substance which prevents and cures scurvy. Although Szent-Györgyi was awarded the 1937 *Nobel Prize in Medicine*, many felt that King was the responsible for its development if not more so.

In 1928 the arctic anthropologist and adventurer Vilhjalmur Stefansson (1879- 1962) attempted to prove his theory of how Eskimo (Inuit) people are able to avoid scurvy with almost no plant food in their diet. This had long been a puzzle because the disease had struck European Arctic explorers living on similar high-meat diets. Stefansson theorised that the native peoples of the Arctic got their vitamin C from fresh meat that was raw or minimally cooked. Starting in February 1928, for one year he and a colleague lived on an animal-flesh-only diet under medical supervision at New York's Bellevue Hospital; they remained healthy.

In 1933-1934, the British chemists Sir Walter Norman Haworth (1883–1950) and Sir Edmund Hirst (1898-1975) and, independently, the Polish Tadeus Reichstein (1897–1996), succeeded in synthesizing the vitamin, the first to be artificially produced. This made possible the cheap mass production of vitamin C. Haworth was awarded the 1937 Nobel Prize in Chemistry largely for this work. The synthetic form of the vitamin is identical to the natural form.

Research directed at the determination of the level of vitamin C necessary to prevent scurvy led to the establishment of a recommended dietary allowance (RDA) for vitamin C of 60 mg per day [7]. And, basically, what most scientists and doctors are taught in their medical training about nutrition is that certain nutrients prevent certain deficiency diseases. There is abundant evidence that this minimal RDA levels of 60 mg in no way reflects the optimal level of vitamin C required for excellent health. In fact, Irwin Stone blames the emphasis of vitamin C as an antiscurvy vitamin rather than an essential nutrient since the 1930's for halting progress of clinical research and therapeutic application of vitamin C for the treatment of a wide number of diseases. During the 1940's and 50's, Dr. Frederick Robert Klenner, (1907 – 1984) pioneered large doses of vitamin C for the treatment of many viral diseases, including poliomyelitis [8-10].

STRUCTURE AND BIOSYNTHESIS OF VITAMIN C

Vitamin C, also known as L-Ascorbic acid, L-xyloascorbic acid, 3-oxo-L-gulofuranolactone (enol form), L-3-ketothreohexuronic acid lactone and antisorbutic vitamin, has the chemical formula C6H8O6 and a molecular weight of 176.12. This 6-carbon molecule is structurally very similar to the sugar D-glucose (Figure 1), a point of significance which will be addressed when considering the mode of action and mechanisms underlying vitamin C's therapeutic effectiveness with diabetes and heart disease. Some microorganisms such as the yeast Saccharomyces cerevistae have been shown to be able to synthesize ascorbic acid.

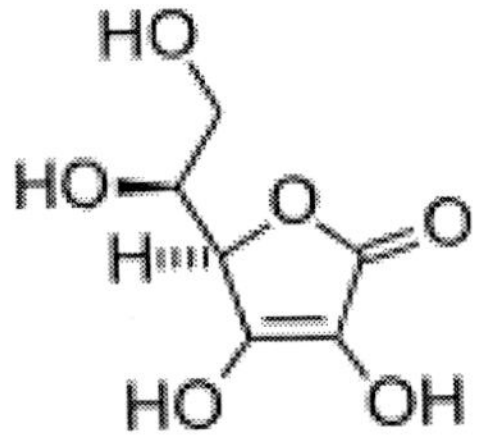

Figure 1. Chemical Structure of Vitamin C.

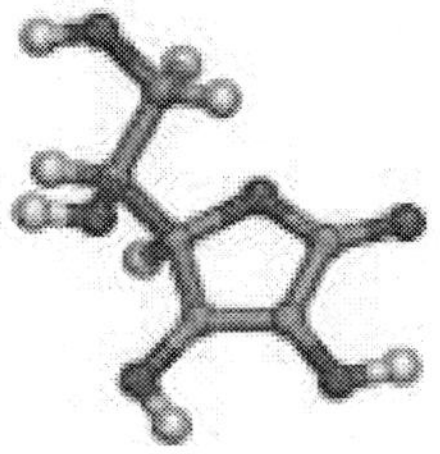

Figure 2. 3 D Representation of vitamin C.

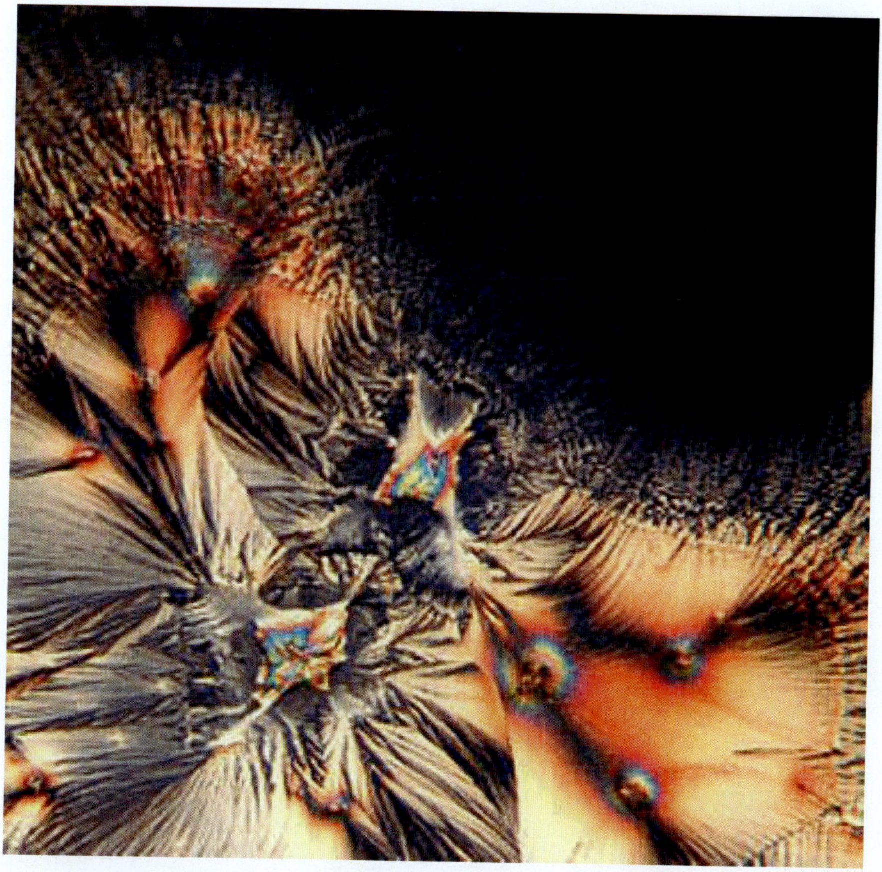

Figure 3. Crystals of Vitamin C.

Humans, non-human primates, guinea pigs, the red-vented bulbul (an Asian bird), the Indian fruit-eating bat, rainbow trout and Coho salmon are the only animal species lacking the complete enzymatic machinery to synthesize vitamin C. It has been shown that humans and guinea pigs lack the enzyme gulonolactone oxidase, which oxidizes l-gulonolactone to 2-keto-l-gulonolactone. This, then, is the 25-60 million year old evolutionary accident spoken of earlier which has deprived humans and these other animals of their ability to synthesize their own vitamin C. Whether, as genetic engineering techniques become more refined in the future, it may become feasible to re-introduce this enzyme back into human cells, must remain a subject beyond the scope of this book, however fascinating and intriguing an idea.

ASCORBATE SALTS

Preparations of vitamin C are frequently obtainable as salts of ascorbic acid, commonly as sodium or calcium ascorbate. Sodium (calcium) ascorbate is prepared from ascorbic acid and sodium (calcium) carbonate by controlled precipitation in dilute acetone or alcohol [11]. Ester-CR ascorbate, prepared totally in aqueous solutions, has not, therefore, been exposed to these toxic chemicals. The more neutral pH and buffering power of ascorbate salts compared with ascorbic acid (AA) is frequently cited as a superior attribute of ascorbate products.

Metabolism, Absorption and Bioavailability

Transport of vitamin C is a saturable and dose dependent process that occurs by active transport. At the intestine and cells AA is oxidized to DHAA, which is more quickly transported across the cell membrane. Once inside the tissue or intestinal epithelium the vitamin is reduced back to AA. The degree of intestinal absorption decreases as intake of AA increases. Intakes of 1 to 1.5 grams results in 50% absorption, but at intakes over 12 grams only 16% of the vitamin is absorbed. In contrast, an intake of less than 20 mg has a 98% absorption rate [12]. Absorption of vitamin C is greater when several individual doses of vitamin C, in quantities less than one gram, are taken throughout the day rather than one megadose [13]. Eighty to ninety-five percent of the vitamin C found in foods is absorbed [12]. Furthermore, the bioavailability of synthetic and "natural" forms of the vitamin differ very little despite the claims made by manufacturers [12, 13]. Vitamin C absorption can be impaired by a number of factors. A single large dose saturates the enzyme kinetics for vitamin C, leading to excess AA in the intestinal lumen, which causes numerous gastrointestinal problems. Pectin and zinc also inhibit AA absorption, but this mechanism is not well understood. A high iron concentration in the gastrointestinal tract may cause oxidative destruction and in turn impair uptake [12].

Transport

Active transport is the main mechanism of vitamin C distribution within the body. Simple diffusion may occur in the mouth and stomach but accounts for only a very small percentage of uptake [12]. Sodium-independent transport systems shuttle vitamin C across the basolateral membrane of the intestinal cells. In the plasma absorbed ascorbic and dehydroascorbate (DHAA) can either be transported freely or be bound to albumin. Ascorbate can also move into body cells and tissues [12]. As previously mentioned DHAA is the primary form of vitamin C that crosses cellular membranes. The adrenal and pituitary glands, red blood cells, lymphocytes, and neutrophils all receive vitamin C in the form of DHAA [12, 13].

Storage

Vitamin C is stored throughout body tissues and blood. Ascorbic acid content of blood components, fluid, and tissue varies widely on an individual basis. Tissue concentrations exceed those found in the plasma by three to ten times. Energy-driven transport pumps are responsible for the higher tissue concentrations of vitamin C versus the plasma. Both tissue and plasma levels of vitamin C are correlated to intake up to 90 mg/day [12]. The total body pool of vitamin C has been estimated, using radio-labeled isotopes, to a maximum of 20 mg/kg body weight. This corresponds to a plasma AA concentration of 57 umol/L. Alternate techniques of measurement have estimated maximum total body AA stores to be 22 mg/kg[13]. The pituitary glands, adrenal glands, and lens of the eye contain the highest vitamin C content (at least140umol/100 g/weight) within the body [12, 13]. In contrast the saliva and plasma have the lowest AA content[13]. Vitamin C content of cardiac tissue is between 28 and 85 ml/100g wet weight, while that in skeletal muscle is approximately 17 ml/100g wet weight [13]. Other tissues with intermediate levels of vitamin C include the kidneys, brain, liver, lungs, and thyroid. The water-soluble properties of vitamin C prevent it from being stored in the adipose tissue of the body.

EXCRETION

The average half-life of AA is believed to be between 16 and 20 days [13]. Its half-life is inversely related to intake. The water-soluble properties of vitamin C lead to urinary excretion of the vitamin. Metabolites of vitamin C including dehydroascorbate (DHAA), oxalic acid, 2-O-methyl ascorbate, and 2-ketoascorbitol are also excreted from the body via the urinary system [12, 13]. The kidneys play a major role in vitamin C excretion and retention. DHAA and AA can be reabsorbed by the kidney tubules as long as body pool levels are equal to or less than 1500 mg. Levels within the body that are 1500 mg or less will result in no urinary excretion of vitamin C [12]. As the level of the pool increase (above 1500 mg) the reabsorption efficiency of the kidneys decrease. Thus, body pool levels from 1500 to 3000 mg relate to tissue saturation of the vitamin [12]. Plasma ascorbate levels between 0.8 and 1.4 mg/dl are considered the renal threshold. Above these levels, vitamin C will be excreted rather than reabsorbed by the kidneys [12].

SOURCES OF VITAMIN C

Vitamin C is obtained through the diet by the vast majority of the world's population. The richest natural sources are fruits and vegetables, and of those, the camu cam fruit and the billygoat plum contain the highest concentration of the vitamin. It is also present in some cuts of meat, especially liver. Vitamin C is the most widely taken nutritional supplement and is available in a variety of forms from tablets and drink mixes to pure ascorbic acid crystals in capsules or as plain powder.

Rose hips are a particularly rich source of vitamin C. Citrus fruits (orange, lemon, grapefruit, lime), tomatoes, and potatoes are good common sources of vitamin C. Other foods that are good sources of vitamin C include papaya, broccoli, Brussels sprouts, black currants, strawberries, cauliflower, spinach, cantaloupe, kiwifruit, cranberries and red peppers.

Emblica officinalis often referred to as Indian gooseberry or amla, is one of the richest known sources of vitamin C (720 mg/100g of fresh pulp or up to 900 mg/100g of pressed juice) – it contains 30 times the amount found in oranges.

The amount of vitamin C in foods of plant origin depends on:

- the precise variety of the plant
- the soil condition
- the climate in which it grew
- the length of time since it was picked
- the storage conditions

- the method of preparation. Cooking in particular is often said to destroy vitamin C - but see the section on Food preparation

FOOD PREPARATION

Vitamin C is highly sensitive to air, water, and temperature. About 25% of the vitamin C in vegetables can be lost simply by blanching (boiling or steaming the food for a few minutes). This same degree of loss occurs in the freezing and unthawing of vegetables and fruits. Cooking of vegetables and fruits for longer periods of time (10-20 minutes) can result in a loss of over one half of the total vitamin C content. When fruits and vegetables are canned and then reheated, only 1/3 of the original vitamin C content may be left. Consumption of vitamin C-rich foods in their fresh, raw form is the best way to maximize vitamin C intake.

Vitamin C enriched teas and infusions have increasingly appeared on supermarket shelves. Such products would be nonsense if boiling temperatures did indeed destroy vitamin C at the rate it had previously been suggested. It should be noted however that as of 2004 most academics not directly involved in vitamin C research still teach that boiling temperatures will destroy vitamin C very rapidly.

It is important to choose a suitable method of food preparation that conserves vitamin C content. When cooking vegetables, one should seek to minimize temperature and duration of cooking and not discard water used in preparation (e.g., by steam cooking or by making soup). Food source vitamin C is identical to that in supplements. The structure of vitamin C is well understood, (see ascorbic acid) and there is no difference in benefit between natural and synthetic forms (although fruits and vegetables contain various other nutrients, and vitamin C is not their only health benefit).

Recent observations suggest that the impact of temperature and cooking on vitamin C may have been overestimated:

Since it is water soluble, vitamin C will strongly leach into the cooking water while cooking most vegetables - but this doesn't necessarily mean the vitamin is destroyed - it's still there, but it's in the cooking water. This may also suggest how the apparent misconception about the extent to which boiling temperatures destroy vitamin C might have been the result of flawed research: If the vitamin C content of vegetables (and not of the water) was measured subsequent to cooking them, then that content would have been much lower, though the vitamin has not actually been destroyed [14-16] .

Not only the temperature, but also the exposure time is significant. Contrary to what was previously and is still commonly assumed, it can take much longer than two or three minutes to destroy vitamin C at boiling point [14-16].

It also appears that cooking doesn't necessarily leach vitamin C in all vegetables at the same rate; it has been suggested that the vitamin is not destroyed when boiling broccoli. This may be a result of vitamin C leaching into the cooking water at a slower rate from this vegetable.

Pregnant and Lactating Women

Pregnant or lactating women also require a higher intake of vitamin C to maintain optimal plasma vitamin C concentrations [17, 18]. The higher requirement is due to active placental vitamin C transport, whereby vitamin C concentrations are significantly higher in cord blood and in newborn infants than in the mothers, and the loss of vitamin C through milk [18, 19]. The current RDA for women during pregnancy and lactation is 85 and 120 mg/day, respectively [20].

Vitamin C in Elderly

The elderly are prone to vitamin C deficiency because of dietary habits [17, 18, 21]. They also appear to have a higher requirement for vitamin C, although the evidence is inconsistent [17]. The RDA for those over 70 years of age is the same as for young adults (75 mg for women and 90 mg for men) [20]. Oxidative processes have been implicated in aging and it has been proposed antioxidants may have beneficial effects on cognitive functions in the elderly [22]. In one cross-sectional study there was no association between cognitive function and intake of vitamin C (>160 mg/day compared with <70 mg/day) [23]. However, two other studies have shown high plasma vitamin C concentrations lower the prevalence of severe cognitive impairment [24, 25].

Deficiency Symptoms of Vitamin C

Full-blown symptoms of the vitamin C deficiency disease called scurvy - including bleeding gums and skin discoloration due to ruptured blood vessels - are rare in the U.S. Poor wound healing, however, is not rare, and can be a symptom of vitamin C deficiency. Weak immune function, including susceptibility to colds and other infections, can also be a telltale sign of vitamin C deficiency. Since the lining of our respiratory tract also depend heavily on vitamin C for protection, respiratory infection and other lung-related conditions can also be symptomatic of vitamin C deficiency.

Vitamin C Dose Recommendations

Some researchers have calculated the amount needed for an adult human to achieve similar blood serum levels as vitamin C synthesizing mammals as follows:

- 400 mg per day – Linus Pauling Institute and US National Institutes of Health (NIH) Recommendation.
- 500 mg twice per day – Professor Roc Ordman's recommendation in free radical research [26].

- 6000-12000 mg per day – Thomas Levy, Colorado Integrative Medical Centre recommendation.
- 6000-18000 mg per day – Linus Pauling's own daily recommendation from 3000 mg to 200,000 mg per day based on a protocol described by Robert Cathcart [26] known as a vitamin C flush wherein escalating doses of vitamin C are given until diarrhea develops, then choosing the highest dose that does not cause diarrhea (bowel tolerance threshold). High doses (thousands of mg) may result in diarrhea, which is harmless if the dose is reduced immediately. Some researchers [27] claim the onset of diarrhea to be an indication of where the body's true vitamin C requirement lies.

Recommendations for vitamin C minimum daily intake dose are difference in various national agencies. UK Food Standards Agency recommendation's is 40 mg per day. U.S. Food and Nutrition Board 2004 recommended daily allowance (RDA) for vitamin C is 60–95 mg per day.

Vitamin C Toxicity

Vitamin C is recognized to be one of the least toxic substances known to medicine. For example, in the rat, the LD_{50} has been reported as 11900 mg/kg. There are very few research studies that document vitamin C toxicity at any level of supplementation, and there are no documented toxic affects whatsoever for vitamin C in relation to food and diet. At high supplemental doses involving 5 or more grams of vitamin C, diarrhea can result from the fluid in the intestine becoming too concentrated. A common symptom of unabsorbed vitamin C left in the gastrointestinal tract is osmotic diarrhea [12].

Large supplemental doses of vitamin C can also increase levels of uric acid in the urine, because vitamin C can be broken down into uric acid. However, it is not clear that increased uric acid in the urine can increase a person's risk of forming uric acid kidney stones.

Finally, vitamin C can increase a person's absorption of iron from plant foods; and persons who have health problems related to excess free iron in their cells may want to consider avoiding high supplemental doses of vitamin C. It is important to remember that all of the above toxicity-related issues involve vitamin C in supplemental form, not as it naturally occurs in food.

In 2000, the National Academy of Sciences set a Tolerable Upper Intake Level (UL) for vitamin C at 2 grams for adults 19 years or older [12].

Potential problems with pharmacological doses may also include "rebound scurvy," which occurs when the intake of high levels is abruptly stopped. In excess states (>4 g/day), high levels of ascorbate and, significantly, one of its metabolites, oxalate, are found in urine and may increase the risk of renal-oxalate stone formation. The latter is pertinent, as it accounts for one of the few potential clinical toxicities of systemic vitamin C supplementation [28].

Clinical Application and Psychiatric Relevance

Machlin [29] divided the history of the vitamins into five periods. The first phase was present from 1500 B.C. to about 1900 A.D. when it was empirically observed that certain foods prevented some diseases. In 1747 it was determined that only the sailors given citrus fruits recovered from scurvy. It wasn't until nearly 200 years later that vitamin C was identified. The second period started about 1890 and continued until about 1910. During this period the relationship between the lack of certain foods and disease became established. The third phase from 1900 to 1948 was the golden age of vitamin discovery, isolation and synthesis of vitamins. The fourth phase from 1933 began with the first commercial synthesis of vitamin C and continues today. These four phases comprise the vitamin-as-prevention paradigm. The fifth phase is the recognition of health effects beyond prevention and new biochemical functions. It is the vitamin-as-treatment paradigm.

For many years it was widely believed that the only function of ascorbate in the body was to promote collagen synthesis and that its only role in therapeutics was to treat scurvy. However, research in the last few years has revealed new important functions for ascorbate in the body, in particular in the brain. Vitamin C is heavily concentrated in the brain, but its exact role in brain function is not understood. There are over 500 references on Medline referring to vitamin C and the brain.

The brain contains the highest level of ascorbate in the body and there are active uptake mechanisms in the choroid plexus and cell membrane to maintain intracellular levels at 16-25 times higher than blood levels. Levels of extracellular brain ascorbate vary greatly according to our activity, being lowest during sleep and highest with prolong activity and stress. The transport proteins that take up glutamate do so in exchange for ascorbate. Thus uptake of glutamate is accompanied by release of ascorbate. Ascorbate modulates activity at glutamate receptors and also protects NMDA receptors against glutamate toxicity [30]. That's data certainly so important in light of modern glutamatergic theory of schizophrenia. Much research was published from the 1942 [31], and recently examined the influence of standard and high dose therapy, as well as short-term or long-term treatment with vitamin C both in combination and as monotherapy.

Vitamin C and Schizophrenia

In the first report by Horwitt in 1942 [31] that schizophrenic patients receiving the usual dietary amounts of ascorbic acid had lower concentrations of ascorbic acid in the blood than people in good health.

In the 1968 Linus Pauling wrote: "The methods principally used now for treating patients with mental disease are psychotherapy (psychoanalysis and related efforts to provide insight and to decrease environmental stress), chemotherapy (mainly with the use of powerful synthetic drugs, such as chlorpromazine, or powerful natural products from plants, such as reserpine), and convulsive shock therapy (electroconvulsive therapy, insulin coma therapy, pentylenetetrazol shock therapy). I have reached the conclusion that another general method of treatment, which may be called orthomolecular therapy, may be found to be of great value, and may turn out to be the best method of treatment for many patients." [32].

There appears to be an inverse correlation between ascorbic acid intake and the risk of schizophrenia [33]. Even when the dietary vitamin C intake is adequate for non-schizophrenics, schizophrenics may have depressed plasma levels and may demonstrate a greatly reduced urinary excretion of ascorbic acid after an ascorbic acid load [34, 35], suggesting that the utilization of vitamin C in schizophrenics may be enhanced. Suboticanec et al. [36], in evaluation schizophrenic patients on the same hospital diet as a control group, was found that the schizophrenic patients had significantly lower levels of fasting plasma vitamin C and 6-hour urinary vitamin C excretion after an ascorbic acid load test. After giving 70 mg of vitamin C daily for 4 weeks, there were no differences in plasma vitamin C levels between the schizophrenic and control subjects, but urinary vitamin C excretion after the vitamin C load test remained significantly lower in schizophrenic patients. Supplementation with 1 g of vitamin C daily for 4 weeks not only eliminated the differences in plasma vitamin C levels, but also increased the urinary vitamin C excretion of schizophrenic patients to the level of the control subjects. This study supports the hypothesis that schizophrenic patients require higher levels of vitamin C than healthy control subjects for optimum vitamin C status.

One of the first significant controlled trials of ascorbic acid in chronic psychiatric patients was reported in 1963 by Milner [37]. This double-blind study was made in 40 chronic male patients: 34 suffered from schizophrenia, 4 had manic-depressive psychosis, and 2 had general paresis. Twenty of the patients, selected at random, received 1 gm of ascorbic acid a day for three weeks; the rest received a placebo. Milner concluded that "statistically significant improvement in the depressive, manic, and paranoid symptoms-complexes, together with an improvement in overall personality functioning, was obtained following saturation with ascorbic acid". He suggested that chronic psychiatric patients would benefit from the administration of ascorbic acid.

Up to 6 grams daily of vitamin C has been reported to be beneficial for people with schizophrenia [38]. In one case the addition of 400 IU daily of vitamin E enhanced this benefit [39]. A small preliminary trial using 8 grams daily of vitamin C showed decreases in hallucinations, suspiciousness, and unusual and disorganized thoughts in 77% of schizophrenic patients [40]. In all reported cases, patients were also being treated with psychiatric medications. Rationale of use the vitamin C in combination with antipsychotic medications that vitamin C is a competitive antagonist at dopamine receptors. Vitamin C antagonized the effect of amphetamines and enhances the effects of antipsychotic drug haloperidol [41]. Dakhale et al. reported that supplementation of vitamin C to atypical antipsychotic reduces oxidative stress and improves the outcome of schizophrenia. Increased serum MDA and decreased plasma ascorbic acid levels researchers found in schizophrenic patients. These levels were reversed significantly after treatment with vitamin C along with atypical antipsychotic compared to placebo with atypical antipsychotic. The Brief Psychiatric Rating Scale (BPRS) change scores at 8 weeks improved statistically significant with vitamin C as compared to placebo. Researches conclusion that oral supplementation of vitamin C with atypical antipsychotic reverses ascorbic acid levels, reduces oxidative stress, and improves the BPRS scores, hence both the drugs in combination can be used in the treatment of schizophrenia [42].

Arvindakshan and coworkers reported that supplementation with a combination of omega-3 fatty acids and antioxidants (vitamins E and C) improves the outcome of schizophrenia [43]. The investigators used supplementation with a mixture of EPA (eicosapentaenoic acid)/DHA (docosahexaenoic acid) (180:120 mg) and antioxidants (vitamin

E/C, 400 IU: 500 mg) orally morning and evening to schizophrenic patients (N=33) for 4 months. The red blood cell (RBC) membrane fatty acid levels, plasma lipid peroxides and clinical measures were carried out by established procedures at pretreatment, posttreatment and after 4 months of postsupplementation period to determine the stability of treatment effects within patients. Levels of fatty acids and lipid peroxides was compared with their levels in normal controls (NC) (N=45). Posttreatment levels of red blood cell (RBC) as essential polyunsaturated fatty acids (EPUFA) were significantly higher than pretreatment levels as well as levels in normal controls without any significant increase in plasma peroxides. Concomitantly, there was significant reduction in psychopathology based on reduction in individual total scores for BPRS and the Positive and Negative Syndrome Scale (PANSS), general psychopathology - PANSS and increase in Henrich's Quality of Life Scale (QOL). The EPUFA levels returned to pretreatment levels after 4 months of supplementation washout. However, the clinical improvement was significantly retained. The rationale for adjunctive use essential fatty acids and their metabolites, such as prostaglandins, have been considered for some time to improve the outcome of schizophrenia [44]. This is based on altered membrane phospholipid composition observed in schizophrenia for over 40 years [35].

Vitamin C and Alzheimer's Disease

The role of oxidative stress in the pathogenesis of disease such Alzheimer's disease has received much attention. Thus, there is considerable interest in the potential contribution of antioxidants to the prevention of this disease. Many researchers founded that vitamin C can be helpful in Alzheimer's disease [45].

Almost of investigation in this area was done with large number of patients with long duration of supplementation. Overwhelmingly of cases vitamin C was use with other vitamins. Gray et al. [46] and Zandi et al. [47] reported that use of vitamin E and vitamin C supplements in combination is associated with reduced prevalence and incidence of AD. Antioxidant supplements merit further study as agents for the primary prevention of AD. Quinn et al. [48] report data from first longitudinal analysis of cerebrospinal fluid (CSF) F2-isoprostanes (IsoPs), quantitative in vivo biomarkers of lipid peroxidation, in patients with mild Alzheimer's disease (AD). CSF F2-IsoPs were significantly increased in patients followed over one year, correlated with some clinical indices of dementia following correction for variation in ventricular enlargement, and were significantly lower in patients who used both alpha-tocopherol and vitamin C.

Steptoe et al. [49] have carried out a randomized trial comparing brief behavioral counseling with nutritional education counseling to increase fruit and vegetable consumption and associated biomarkers in adults from a low-income neighborhood. Investigators reported that individual differences in improvements in physical health status and self-rated health were correlated with increases in fruit and vegetable intake and in plasma vitamins C and E, independently of age, gender, ethnicity, financial status, smoking, BMI and use of vitamin supplements. They conclude that participation was associated with improved health-related quality of life. Increases in fruit and vegetable intake and plasma vitamin levels may stimulate beneficial changes in physical health status in socio-economically deprived adults.

In other study 5395 participants who, at baseline (1990-1993), were aged at least 55 years, free of dementia and noninstitutionalized and had reliable dietary assessment was investigated [50]. Participants were reexamined in 1993-1994 and 1997-1999 and were continuously monitored for incident dementia. Researchers founded that incidence of Alzheimer disease associated with dietary intake of beta carotene, flavonoids, vitamin C, and vitamin E. They conclusion was that high dietary intake of vitamin C and vitamin E may lower the risk of Alzheimer disease. Similar results reported by Riviere et al. [51].

Vitamin C and Affective Disorders

Vitamin C has many functions: it can function as a coenzyme or as a cofactor in the body. It appears to be necessary for the normal function of cellular units and subcellular structures. In metabolism, vitamin C functions to accept and donate hydrogen. Vitamin C is important and necessary for the synthesis of the neurotransmitters, norepinephrine and serotonin. It catalyzes the conversion of dopamine to norepinephrine and the conversion of tryptophan to serotonin.

Vitamin C, as the cofactor for tryptophan-5-hydroxylase, catalyzes the hydroxylation of tryptophan to serotonin [52]. Vitamin C may be valuable for patients with depression associated with low levels of serotonin. In one study, 40 chronic psychiatric inpatients received 1 g/day of ascorbic acid or placebo for three weeks, in double-blind fashion. In the vitamin C group, significant improvements were seen in depressive, manic and paranoid symptom complexes, as well as in overall functioning [37]. Vitamin C supplementation may be therefore helpful for depression as it may decrease levels of the trace mineral vanadium in the body. Raised levels of vanadium have been found in the blood plasma and hair of individuals with depression [53].

Supplementation with vitamin C associated not only with mood elevation as well as increases intercourse frequency. In one study was found that vitamin C supplementation by modulates catecholaminergic activity, decreases stress reactivity, approach anxiety and prolactin release, improves vascular function, and increases oxytocin release. All these processes are relevant to sexual behavior and mood. In randomized double-blind, placebo-controlled 14 day trial of sustained-release ascorbic acid (AA) (42 healthy young adults; 3000 mg/day) and placebo (39 healthy young adults), subjects with partners recorded penile-vaginal intercourse (FSI), noncoital partner sex, and masturbation in daily diaries, and also completed the Beck Depression Inventory before and after the trial. The AA group reported greater FSI frequency, an effect most prominent in subjects not cohabiting with their sexual partner, and in women. The AA but not placebo group also experienced a decrease in Beck Depression scores [54].

Few intervention studies examined the effects of selective serotonin re-uptake inhibitors, on lipid peroxidation, superoxide dismutase (SOD) activity and AA concentrations. There was a significant increase in serum SOD, serum malonyldialdehyde (MDA) and decrease in plasma ascorbic acid levels in patients of major depression as compared to control subjects. The trend reversed significantly after treatment with fluoxetine and citalopram and results indicate a greater reduction in oxidative stress with citalopram than fluoxetine [55].

Some healthcare professionals recommend vitamin C to reduce the symptom of dry mouth, a side effect experienced by many people taking antidepressant medications.

VITAMIN C AND OTHER PSYCHIATRIC DISORDERS

Few intervention studies with AA supplementation for conditions such as autism [56-60], attention deficit hyperactivity disorder (ADHD) [61], Down's syndrome [62] and anxiety disorder have reported.

Has vitamin C been used in the treatment of autism? Only two studies in which vitamin C was specifically evaluated as an intervention in autism we found. The first study reports that AA is of benefit in autism if a dose ranges from 1 to 3 grams per day of vitamin C is used. [63]. In the second, 30-week's, double-blind, placebo-controlled trial scientist's have studied the effectiveness of ascorbic acid as a supplemental pharmacological treatment for autistic children in residential treatment. In the last study the dose range was significantly higher - 8g/70kg/day [60]. In this study residential school children were randomly assigned to either ascorbate-ascorbate-placebo treatment order group or ascorbate-placebo-ascorbate treatment order group. Each treatment phase lasted 10 weeks and behaviors were rated weekly using the Ritvo-Freeman scale. The investigators reported significant group by phase interactions were found for total scores and also sensory motor scores indicating a reduction in symptom severity associated with the ascorbic acid treatment.

Another clinical area where brain ascorbate and other anti oxidants and nutrition may be relevant is Down's syndrome. Individuals with Down's syndrome have signs of possible brain damage prior to birth. Some of the cognitive impairments are likely due to post-natal hydrogen peroxide-mediated oxidative stress caused by overexpression of the superoxide dismutase (SOD-1) gene, which is located on the triplicated 21st chromosome and known to be 50% overexpressed. Thiel et al. [62] in their paper suggest that essential nutrients such as folate, vitamin B_6, vitamin C, vitamin E, selenium, and zinc, as well as alpha-lipoic acid and carnosine may possibly be partially preventive. This paper hypothesizes that nutritional factors begun prenatally, in early infancy, or later may prevent or delay the onset of dementia in the Down syndrome population.

There are some anecdotal reports regarding improvement of the outcome of ADHD after vitamin C supplementation [61]. This is the first study to show that supplementation with flax oil-based ω- 3 precursors in combination with antioxidants is effective in significantly improving symptoms of ADHD such as impulsivity, restlessness, inattention and self control. Pre- and post – supplementation hyperactivity scores showed statistically significant improvement. Although the results of this study are encouraging, the limitation of the trial was a lack of placebo group.

A study measuring possible brain and central-nervous-system stimulants and sedatives demonstrated that vitamin C has potent sedative, antianxiety properties. In large doses, vitamin C can have a powerful tranquilizing effect and is known to decrease anxiety.

One of the studies showed significantly decreased levels of anxiety among a group of alcoholics treated with megavitamins [64]. In this study over a twenty-one-day period, the group took approximately three grams of vitamin C, three grams of niacin, six hundred milligrams of B_6, and six hundred international units (IU) of vitamin E per day. A comparison group received only inert gelatin capsules. None of the subjects in either group took antidepressants or anti-anxiety drugs. Anxiety levels in both groups were measured three times over the twenty-one days. They fell dramatically only in the group on megavitamin therapy. Vitamin C also promotes restful sleep.

DISCUSSION

For few last decades vitamin C, some other vitamins and nutrients have established a significant place in both general medicine and psychiatry. Many investigators have reported their results with vitamin C supplementation for treatment of many psychiatric conditions – affective disorder, anxiety, schizophrenia, autism, Down's syndrome, Alzheimer disease, ADHD and others [60-62]. Same studies have found correlation between vitamin C plasma level and psychiatric conditions. As we have already mentioned, vitamin C is involved and plays an important role in the biochemical and biosynthesis process of some neurotransmitters and enzymes.

The idea of using vitamins to treat schizophrenia was based on the theoretical assumption of their antioxidant's properties. There is increasing evidence from many different directions that, in schizophrenia, nerve and other cells are oxidized more readily than usual. This suggests an increased need for antioxidant intakes which are higher than those provided by ordinary multivitamin and multimineral tablets.

Data analysis of overwhelmingly investigations showed that preferably use vitamin C with other vitamins and /or nutrients and not along, especially with vitamin E [39, 43, 44]. It is important to use two antioxidants, one which will work in the watery parts of the body – water soluble antioxidant, and one which will work in the cell membranes – lipid soluble antioxidant. The principle water soluble antioxidants in the body are ascorbate and glutathione. The principle lipid soluble antioxidant are vitamin E and variety of carotens, which are relatives of vitamin A. Vitamin C works best in the watery parts of the body and vitamin E in the cell membranes. Together they produce a coordinated effect. When vitamin E neutralizes a toxic reactive oxygen species it is oxidized itself. The conversion of this oxidized vitamin E back to the reduced form is carried out by vitamin C or by glutathione [41].

Vitamin E was used for treatment tardive dyskinesia caused by antipsychotic treatment, but pharmacologists warn against high dosage of vitamin E because of its pro-oxidative effects on low-density lipoprotein with consecutive cardiac risks. Addition of vitamin C probably reduces this risk because of its interactions with vitamin E, i.e. vitamin C reduces vitamin E radicals formed when vitamin E scavenges the oxygen radicals. Michael and coworkers tested the safety and efficacy of combining vitamins C and E in a sample of patients with affective disorders and tardive dyskinesia who had previously been treated with antipsychotics due to psychotic symptoms. In all 6 patients, a reduction of tardive symptoms was seen, but the mechanisms by which vitamin C and E attenuates the symptoms of tardive dyskinesia are not completely understood [65].

It is important to mention that there are works that showed that dopamine activity was antagonized to vitamin C. Indeed its activity is similar to antipsychotic medications. In addition to antagonized activity on dopamine resorts, it was found that vitamin C activates as a modulator of glutamate receptor. All the above suggests that vitamin C is essential in treating schizophrenia patients. Indeed, there is no consensus about vitamin C dosages. The dosage range moves between tens mg. per day to 6 g per day.

However, a reasonable proposal in the light of current knowledge is that around 500 mg/day of vitamin C and 100 IU of vitamin E should be taken in addition to the multinutrients.

An analysis of information reaches the conclusion that schizophrenia patients can benefit from addition of vitamin C to their daily diet. Indeed there is a need to continue investigating vitamin C ways of influence and involvement in this schizophrenic process and its treatment.

However, we are not found double blind controlled study with large populations that find evidence of a statistically significant therapeutic effect of vitamin C on psychotic symptoms in the patients suffering from resistant schizophrenia or other disorders from schizophrenic spectrum.

Age related diseases, especially Alzheimer's disease are the only area that controlled research on large populations can be found.

Mostly part of researchers' conclusion that high dietary intake of vitamin C and vitamin E may lower the risk of Alzheimer's disease.

Conclusions

Few studies were performed on comparatively large groups of patients. The mostly of studies, except studies with Alzheimer's disease patients, had important limitations, including lack of a control group and double-blind protocol, small number of patients and inclusion of patients who were not very severely pathology. However, further investigation is clearly warranted.

In conclusion the vitamin C is not a replacement for those other approaches. Vitamin C and other vitamin's supplementation is a way of putting the biochemistry of the brain in the best possible shape to allow other treatments to work. Our attitude towards nutrition must be like a partner in the therapeutic alliance.

References

[1] Klenner FR. Virus pneumonia and its treatment with vitamin C. *South Med. Surg*. 1948; 110: 34-46.

[2] Klenner FR. The treatment of poliomyelitis and other virus diseases with vitamin C. *South Med. Surg*. 1949; 111: 209-214.

[3] Klenner FR. Massive doses of vitamin C and the virus diseases. *South Med. Surg*. 1951; 113: 101-107.

[4] Klenner FR. The vitamin and massage treatment for acute poliomyelitis. *South Med. Surg* 1952; 114: 194-197.

[5] Klenner FR. The use of vitamin C as an antibiotic. *J. Applied Nutr*. 1953; 6.

[6] Klenner FR. The folly in the continued use of a killed polio virus vaccine. *Tri-State Med. J*. 1959: 1-8.

[7] Recommended Dietary Allowances. National Academy of Sciences. Washington: Nat. Acad. Press, 1978.

[8] Waugh WA, King CG. Isolation and identification of vitamin C. J. Biol. Chem. 1932; 97: 325-331.

[9] Szent-Gyorgyi A. Studies on Biological Oxidation and Some of Its Catalysts. Szeged, 1937.

[10] Stone I. The Healing Factor. Vitamin C against Disease: Grosset and Dunlap, 1972.

[11] Stone N, Meister A. Function of ascorbic acid in the conversion of proline to collagen hydroxyproline. *Nature* 1962; 194: 555-7.

[12] Groff JL, Gropper SS, Hunt SM. The Water Soluble Vitamins. Advanced Nutrition and Human Metabolism. Minneapolis: West Publishing Company, 1995; 222-237.

[13] Jacob RA. Vitamin C. In: Shils ME, Olson JA, Shike M, et al., eds. Modern Nutrition in Health and Disease, 9th ed. Baltimore, MD: Williams and Wilkins, 1999; 448-467.

[14] Navarra T, Shankin-Cohen W. The A to Z of Vitamins, Minerals and Supplements (A to Z Encyclopedias), 2nd ed. NY: Checkmark Books, 2006.

[15] Somer E. Essential Guide to Vitamins and Minerals, 2nd ed. New York: Harper Collins Pub Inc, 1996.

[16] Herbert V. Vitamins World Book Encyclopedia, 1999.

[17] Plodin NW. Vitamin C. Pharmacology of micronutrients. New York: Alan R Liss Inc, 1988; 201-244.

[18] Burri BJ, Jacob RA. Human metabolism and the requirement for vitamin C. In: Packer L,Fuchs J, eds. Vitamin C in Health and Disease. New York: Marcel Dekker Inc, 1997; 341-366.

[19] Berger TM, Rifai N, Avery ME, Frei B. Vitamin C in premature and full-term human neonates. *Redox Rep.* 1996; 2: 257-262.

[20] Standing Committee on the Scientific Evaluation of Dietary Reference Intakes, Food and Nutrition Board. Dietary Reference Intakes for Vitamin C, Vitamin E, Selenium, and Beta-carotene, and Other Carotenoids. Washington, DC: National Academy Press, 2000.

[21] Weber P, Bendich A, Schalch W. Vitamin C and human health--a review of recent data relevant to human requirements. *Int. J. Vitam. Nutr. Res.* 1996; 66: 19-30.

[22] Ames BN, Shigenaga MK, Hagen TM. Oxidants, antioxidants, and the degenerative diseases of aging. *Proc. Natl. Acad. Sci. USA* 1993; 90: 7915-22.

[23] Jama JW, Launer LJ, Witteman JC, den Breeijen JH, Breteler MM, Grobbee DE, Hofman A. Dietary antioxidants and cognitive function in a population-based sample of older persons. The Rotterdam Study. *Am. J. Epidemiol.* 1996; 144: 275-80.

[24] Perrig WJ, Perrig P, Stahelin HB. The relation between antioxidants and memory performance in the old and very old. *J. Am. Geriatr. Soc.* 1997; 45: 718-24.

[25] Paleologos M, Cumming RG, Lazarus R. Cohort study of vitamin C intake and cognitive impairment. *Am. J. Epidemiol.* 1998; 148: 45-50.

[26] Cathcart RF. Vitamin C, titrating to bowel tolerance, anascorbemia, and acute induced scurvy. *Med. Hypotheses* 1981; 7: 1359-76.

[27] King G, Beins M, Larkin J, Summers B, Ordman AB. Rate of excretion of vitamin C in human urine Age 1994; 17: 87-92.

[28] Bsoul SA, Terezhalmy GT. Vitamin C in health and disease. *J. Contemp. Dent. Pract.* 2004; 5: 1-13.

[29] Machlin LJ. Beyond deficiency. New views on the function and health effects of vitamins. Introduction. *Ann. N Y Acad. Sci.* 1992; 669: 1-6.

[30] Rebec GV, Pierce RC. A vitamin as neuromodulator: ascorbate release into the extracellular fluid of the brain regulates dopaminergic and glutamatergic transmission. *Prog. Neurobiol.* 1994; 43: 537-65.

[31] Horwitt MK. Ascorbic acid requirements of individuals in a large institution. *Proc. Soc. Exp. Biol. Med.* 1942; 49: 248-250.

[32] Pauling L. Orthomolecular psychiatry. Varying the concentrations of substances normally present in the human body may control mental disease. *Science* 1968; 160: 265-71.

[33] Greenblatt JM, Huffman LC, Reiss AL. Folic acid in neurodevelopment and child psychiatry. *Prog. Neuropsychopharmacol. Biol. Psychiatry* 1994; 18: 647-60.

[34] Godfrey PS, Toone BK, Carney MW, Flynn TG, Bottiglieri T, Laundy M, Chanarin I, Reynolds EH. Enhancement of recovery from psychiatric illness by methylfolate. *Lancet* 1990; 336: 392-5.

[35] Horrobin DF. The membrane phospholipid hypothesis as a biochemical basis for the neurodevelopmental concept of schizophrenia. *Schizophr. Res.* 1998; 30: 193-208.

[36] Suboticanec K, Folnegovic-Smalc V, Korbar M, Mestrovic B, Buzina R. Vitamin C status in chronic schizophrenia. *Biol. Psychiatry* 1990; 28: 959-66.

[37] Milner G. Ascorbic acid in chronic psychiatric patients: a controlled trial. *Br. J. Psychiatry* 1963; 109: 294-299.

[38] Sandyk R, Kanofsky JD. Vitamin C in the treatment of schizophrenia. *Int. J. Neurosci.* 1993; 68: 67-71.

[39] Kanofsky JD, Sandyk R. Antioxidants in the treatment of schizophrenia. *Int. J. Neurosci.* 1992; 62: 97-100.

[40] Beauclair L, Vinogradov S, Riney SJ, Csernansky JG, Hollister LE. An adjunctive role for ascorbic acid in the treatment of schizophrenia? J Clin Psychopharmacol 1987; 7: 282-3.

[41] Smythies JR. The role of ascorbate in brain: therapeutic implications. *J. R Soc. Med.* 1996; 89: 241.

[42] Dakhale GN, Khanzode SD, Khanzode SS, Saoji A. Supplementation of vitamin C with atypical antipsychotics reduces oxidative stress and improves the outcome of schizophrenia. *Psychopharmacology* (Berl) 2005; 182: 494-8.

[43] Arvindakshan M, Ghate M, Ranjekar PK, Evans DR, Mahadik SP. Supplementation with a combination of omega-3 fatty acids and antioxidants (vitamins E and C) improves the outcome of schizophrenia. *Schizophr. Res.* 2003; 62: 195-204.

[44] Peet M, Brind J, Ramchand CN, Shah S, Vankar GK. Two double-blind placebo-controlled pilot studies of eicosapentaenoic acid in the treatment of schizophrenia. *Schizophr. Res.* 2001; 49: 243-51.

[45] Agbayewa MO, Bruce VM, Siemens V. Pyridoxine, ascorbic acid and thiamine in Alzheimer and comparison subjects. *Can. J. Psychiatry.* Revue Canadienne De Psychiatrie 1992; 37: 661-2.

[46] Gray SL, Hanlon JT, Landerman LR, Artz M, Schmader KE, Fillenbaum GG. Is antioxidant use protective of cognitive function in the community-dwelling elderly? *Am. J. Geriatr. Pharmacother.* 2003; 1: 3-10.

[47] Zandi PP, Anthony JC, Khachaturian AS, Stone SV, Gustafson D, Tschanz JT, Norton MC, Welsh-Bohmer KA, Breitner JC. Reduced risk of Alzheimer disease in users of antioxidant vitamin supplements: the Cache County Study. *Arch Neurol.* 2004; 61: 82-8.
[48] Quinn JF, Montine KS, Moore M, Morrow JD, Kaye JA, Montine TJ. Suppression of longitudinal increase in CSF F2-isoprostanes in Alzheimer's disease. *J. Alzheimers Dis.* 2004; 6: 93-7.
[49] Steptoe A, Perkins-Porras L, Hilton S, Rink E, Cappuccio FP. Quality of life and self-rated health in relation to changes in fruit and vegetable intake and in plasma vitamins C and E in a randomised trial of behavioural and nutritional education counselling. *Br. J. Nutr.* 2004; 92: 177-84.
[50] Engelhart MJ, Geerlings MI, Ruitenberg A, van Swieten JC, Hofman A, Witteman JC, Breteler MM. Dietary intake of antioxidants and risk of Alzheimer disease. *Jama* 2002; 287: 3223-9.
[51] Riviere S, Birlouez-Aragon I, Nourhashemi F, Vellas B. Low plasma vitamin C in Alzheimer patients despite an adequate diet. *Int. J. Geriatr. Psychiatry* 1998; 13: 749-54.
[52] Cooper JR. The role of ascorbic acid in the oxidation of tryptophan to 5-hydroxytryptophan. *Ann. N Y Acad. Sci.* 1961; 92: 208-11.
[53] Naylor GJ. Vanadium and manic depressive psychosis. Nutr Health 1984; 3: 79-85.
[54] Brody S. High-dose ascorbic acid increases intercourse frequency and improves mood: a randomized controlled clinical trial. *Biol. Psychiatry* 2002; 52: 371-4.
[55] Khanzode SD, Dakhale GN, Khanzode SS, Saoji A, Palasodkar R. Oxidative damage and major depression: the potential antioxidant action of selective serotonin re-uptake inhibitors. *Redox. Rep.* 2003; 8: 365-70.
[56] Rimland B, Callaway E, Dreyfus P. The effect of high doses of vitamin B6 on autistic children: a double-blind crossover study. *Am. J. Psychiatry* 1978; 135: 472-5.
[57] Lelord G, Muh JP, Barthelemy C, Martineau J, Garreau B, Callaway E. Effects of pyridoxine and magnesium on autistic symptoms--initial observations. *J. Autism. Dev. Disord.* 1981; 11: 219-30.
[58] Martineau J, Barthelemy C, Lelord G. Long-term effects of combined vitamin B6-magnesium administration in an autistic child. *Biological Psychiatry* 1986; 21: 511-8.
[59] Martineau J, Barthelemy C, Garreau B, Lelord G. Vitamin B6, magnesium, and combined B6-Mg: therapeutic effects in childhood autism. *Biological Psychiatry* 1985; 20: 467-78.
[60] Dolske MC, Spollen J, McKay S, Lancashire E, Tolbert L. A preliminary trial of ascorbic acid as supplemental therapy for autism. *Prog. Neuropsychopharmacol. Biol. Psychiatry* 1993; 17: 765-74.
[61] Joshi K, Lad S, Kale M, Patwardhan B, Mahadik SP, Patni B, Chaudhary A, Bhave S, Pandit A. Supplementation with flax oil and vitamin C improves the outcome of Attention Deficit Hyperactivity Disorder (ADHD). Prostaglandins Leukot Essent Fatty Acids 2006; 74: 17-21.
[62] Thiel R, Fowkes SW. Can cognitive deterioration associated with Down syndrome be reduced? *Med. Hypotheses* 2005; 64: 524-32.
[63] Rimland B. Has vitamin C been used in the treatment of autism? Autism Research Review International 1998; 12: 3.

[64] Replogle WH, Eicke FJ. Megavitamin therapy in the reduction of anxiety and depression among alcoholics. *J. Orthomolec. Med.* 1988; 4: 221-224.

[65] Michael N, Sourgens H, Arolt V, Erfurth A. Severe tardive dyskinesia in affective disorders: treatment with vitamin E and C. *Neuropsychobiology* 2002; 46 Suppl 1: 28-30.

In: New Hope for Mental Disturbances
Editors: Vladimir Lerner and Chanoch Meodownik
ISBN 978-1-60692-691-8

Chapter 2

VITAMIN B_6 AS TREATMENT OF PSYCHOTROPIC DRUG-INDUCED MOVEMENT DISORDERS AND ADD-ON TREATMENT OF SCHIZOPHRENIA

Vladimir Lerner[1] and Chanoch Miodownik

[1] Division of Psychiatry, Ministry of Health, Be'er Sheva Mental Health Center, Faculty of Health Sciences, Ben Gurion University of the Negev, Be'er-Sheva, Israel

ABSTRACT

Vitamin B_6 gained immense significance with the discovery in the 1940s of its important role in animal and human nutrition. It is involved in about 100 enzymatic reactions in the body. The most important of these are transamination, decarboxylation, cleavage reactions, substance synthesis, transsulfhydration, desulfhydration, and racemization. Vitamin B_6 deficiency causes a broad spectrum of both physical and mental symptoms. The aims of this chapter were to summarize contemporary data concerning 1) vitamin B_6 and psychotic symptoms; 2) its influence on homocysteine serum level; and 3) vitamin B_6 use for psychotropic drug-induced movement disorders. The data cumulated to date demonstrate that vitamin B_6 may be effective in treating psychotropic drug-induced movement disorders, as in the case of acute movement disturbances as well as tardive movement disorders. The influence on psychotic symptoms was not confirmed, and further studies with higher doses of the vitamin are indicated.

"Megavitamin treatment does not work magically, overnight, like drugs."
— *Dr. Abram Hoffer*

[1] Corresponding author: Vladimir Lerner, Faculty of Health Sciences, Ben Gurion University of the Negev and Psychiatric Department at Be'er Sheva Mental Health Center. Mailing address: Be'er Sheva Mental Health Center, PO Box 4600, Be'er Sheva 84170, Israel. Tel.: +972 8 6401408; Fax: +972 8 6401491; Email: lernervld@yahoo.com.

INTRODUCTION

Vitamin B_6 was discovered in 1926 almost as a by-product of the studies on pellagra. Pellagra is a disease caused by the absence or deficiency of niacin. Hungarian scientist Paul Gyorgy (1893–1976) demonstrated that rats with pellagra were treated by combination vitamins, a mixture known in those days as conventional treatment in pellagra. Unfortunately, the rats were not cured. This clinical problem remained until Paul Gyorgy, who worked at Heidelberg University (Germany), found that there is another essential substance capable of curing a characteristic skin disease in rats (dermatitis acrodynia). The factor was then called the rat anti-acrodynia factor, a deficiency of which causes the so-called 'rat-pellagra'. This substance was called "adermin" [1]. Later it was discovered that vitamin B_6 deficiency may cause niacin deficiency as a result of impaired tryptophan metabolism [2, 3]. In 1939, American researchers gave it the name that now stands – "pyridoxine." This name was a result of its chemical structure — a pyridine ring (5 carbons and 1 nitrogen) and 3 hydroxyl groups — 2-methyl, 3-hydroxy, 5-hydroxymethyl-pyridine. The name pyridoxine has been used as a generic term, especially in the clinical context. Most commercial labels list it as "pyridoxine hydrochloride."

In 1938, Samuel Lepkovsky (1899–1984) reported on the isolation of pure crystalline vitamin B_6. Independently, but slightly later, several other groups of researchers also reported the isolation of crystallized vitamin B_6 [4].

Vitamin B_6 gained immense significance with the discovery in the 1940s of its important role in animal and human nutrition.

Vitamin B_6 is present in the human body as six vitamers, which all share a 2-methyl-3-hydroxypyridine structure but differ in the nature of the C4 and C5 substituents [5].

These compounds are metabolically interchangeable, namely pyridoxine or pyridoxol (the alcohol) (Figure 2), pyridoxal (the aldehyde) (Figure 3) and pyridoxamine (the amine) (Figure 4). All three of these C4 variants can exist with the C5 substituent as a hydroxymethyl group or with this group esterified to phosphate (e.g. pyridoxal 5′-phosphate). In plants the C5 hydroxymethyl group of pyridoxine can be esterified to glucose, forming pyridoxine-5'-β-D-glucoside [6].

The two B_6 vitamers that have been used therapeutically are pyridoxine (hydrochloride) and pyridoxal 5′-phosphate (PLP).

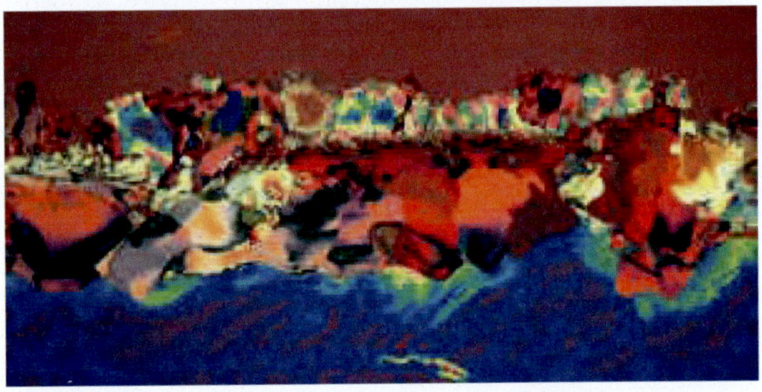

Figure 1. Vitamin B_6 crystals.

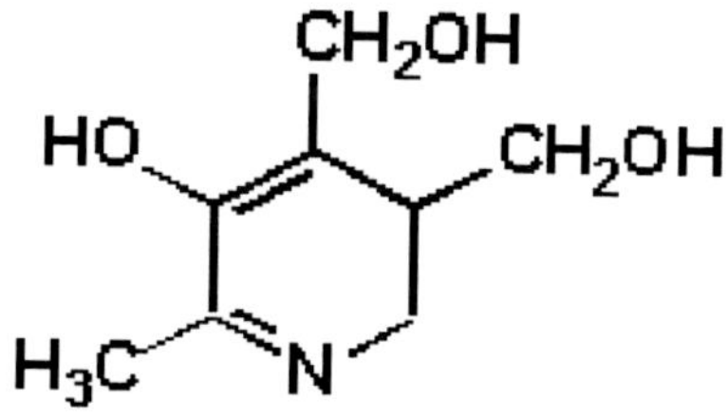

Figure 2. Structure of pyridoxine.

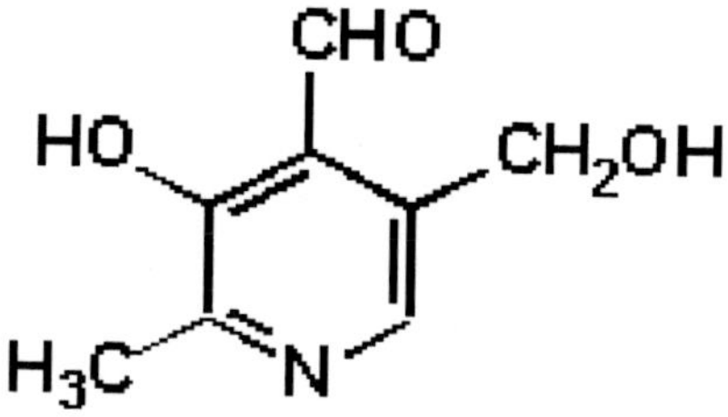

Figure 3. Structure of pyridoxal.

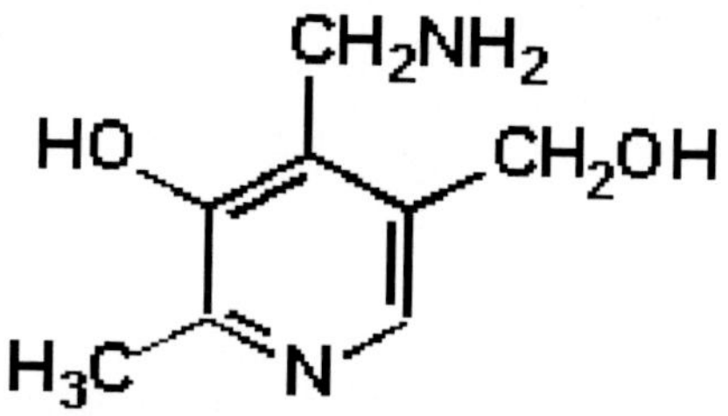

Figure 4. Structure of pyridoxamine.

NATURAL SOURCES OF VITAMIN B_6

Vitamin B_6 is mainly bound to protein in food. Pyridoxine is found especially in plants, whereas pyridoxal and pyridoxamine are principally found in animal tissues. Excellent sources of pyridoxine are chicken, turkey, beef liver, pork, calf and eggs. Good sources include ham and fish (tuna, trout, halibut, herring, salmon), nuts (peanuts, walnuts), bread, corn and whole grain cereals. Generally, vegetables and fruits are rather poor sources of vitamin B_6, although there are products in these food classes that contain considerable amounts of pyridoxine, such as beans and cauliflower, bananas and raisins [7]. The basic sources of vitamin B_6 and each element's daily value are presented in Table 1.

Man and other primates depend on external sources to cover their vitamin B_6 requirements. The Recommended Dietary Allowance (RDA) is the average daily dietary intake level that is sufficient to meet the nutrient requirements of nearly all (97 to 98 percent) healthy individuals in each life-stage, gender, and risk group. For adult males, the RDA is currently 2.2 mg, and for adult women it is 2.0 mg. An addition of 0.6 mg vitamin B_6 per day is suggested in pregnancy. During lactation, an addition of 0.5 mg per day is recommended to provide a level of the vitamin in milk (0.1–0.25 mg/L) that is adequate for the breast-fed infant [8].

Negligible amounts of the vitamin can be synthesized by intestinal bacteria. It is important to know that the vitamin is relatively stable to heat, but it is decomposed by oxidation and ultraviolet light and by an alkaline environment. Freezing of vegetables causes a reduction of up to 25%, and milling of cereals leads to wastes as high as 90%. The cooking losses of processed foods may reach 40%. Vitamin B_6 is easily destroyed by the heavy use of alcohol, drugs or refined sugars [9, 10].

Table 1. Food Sources of Vitamin B_6 [11]

Food	Milligrams (mg) per serving	% DV*
Ready-to-eat cereal, 100% fortified, ¾ c	2.00	100
Potato, baked, flesh and skin, 1 medium	0.70	35
Banana, raw, 1 medium	0.68	34
Garbanzo beans, canned, ½ c	0.57	30
Chicken breast, meat only, cooked, ½ breast	0.52	25
Ready-to-eat cereal, 25% fortified, ¾ c	0.50	25
Oatmeal, instant, fortified, 1 packet	0.42	20
Pork loin, lean only, cooked, 3 oz	0.42	20
Roast beef, eye of round, lean only, cooked, 3 oz	0.32	15
Trout, rainbow, cooked, 3 oz	0.29	15
Sunflower seeds, kernels, dry roasted, 1 oz	0.23	10
Spinach, frozen, cooked, ½ c	0.14	8
Tomato juice, canned, 6 oz	0.20	10
Avocado, raw, sliced, ½ cup	0.20	10
Salmon, sockeye, cooked, 3 oz	0.19	10
Tuna, canned in water, drained solids, 3 oz	0.18	10
Wheat bran, crude or unprocessed, ¼ c	0.18	10
Peanut butter, smooth, 2 tbs.	0.15	8
Walnuts, English/Persian, 1 oz	0.15	8
Soybeans, green, boiled, drained, ½ c	0.05	2
Lima beans, frozen, cooked, drained, ½ c	0.10	6

* DV = Daily Value. DVs are reference numbers based on the Recommended Dietary Allowance (RDA). They were developed to help consumers determine if a food contains a lot or a little of a specific nutrient. The DV for vitamin B_6 is 2.0 milligrams (mg). The percent DV (%DV) listed on the nutrition facts panel of food labels tells you what percentage of the DV is provided in one serving. Percent DVs are based on a 2,000 calorie diet. Your Daily Values may be higher or lower depending on your caloric needs. Foods that provide lower percentages of the DV also contribute to a healthful diet.

BODY STORES

Vitamin B_6 is absorbed in the jejunum through nonsaturable, passive diffusion of the nonphosphorylated forms [12]. It is readily and completely absorbed, although blood levels tend to be low and storage in the body very limited. The storage capacity of the water-soluble vitamins is in general low compared to that of the fat-soluble ones. Small quantities of pyridoxine are widely distributed in body tissues, mainly as pyridoxal-5-phosphate (PLP) in muscles. PLP is the metabolically active coenzyme form of vitamin B_6; it is tightly bound to the proteins albumin and hemoglobin in plasma and red blood cells [8].

Measurement

There are several methods used to assess a person's vitamin B_6 status.They include direct measurement of B_6 vitamers in blood and/or urine or by indicators based on the biochemical function of vitamin B_6 [12-15]. The most commonly used direct measure of vitamin B_6 status is the concentration of pyridoxal-5′-phosphate (PLP) in plasma, which can be readily measured by high performance liquid chromatography (HPLC) or enzymatic methods.

Plasma PLP concentration has been shown to correlate with vitamin B_6 intake in controlled human studies [12, 14, 16, 17]. According to the American Society for Nutritional Sciences, it has been considered that a plasma PLP concentration of more than 30 nmol/L indicates an adequate status in human adults [12, 14], whereas a concentration greater than 20 nmol/L has been used as a more conservative cutoff value [15]. The adequate level of total plasma vitamin B_6 should be greater than 40 nmol/L; adult urinalysis of 4-pyridoxic acid is considered adequate when it is higher than 3 μmol/d, while the total urinary vitamin B_6 level is more than 0.5 μmol/d [14].

If the 20 nmol/L cutoff is used, we recommend that values in the range of 20 to 30 nmol/L be interpreted as indicative of marginal status.

ANTAGONISM AND SYNERGISM

Pyridoxine is sensitive to sunlight. The serum concentration of vitamin B_6 can be influenced by some other drugs. There are more than 40 drugs that interfere with vitamin B_6. The influence may be bi-directional. There are medications that cause elevation of serum level, and they are called synergistic agents. This drug group includes some vitamins from the B family such as niacin, riboflavin, and biotin. Niacin and riboflavin are needed for the interconversion of the different forms of vitamin B_6. On the other hand, there are a few agents that could cause a decreased availability and poor vitamin B_6 status. This group includes anti-tuberculosis drugs (isoniazid and cycloserine), monoamine oxidase inhibitors (phenelzine and tranylcypramine), penicillamine, cyclosporine, pyrazinamide, and tetracyclines. Carbamazepine leads to significant lower PLP levels [18]. The asthma drug theophylline interferes with PLP production by inhibition of pyridoxal kinase [19]. The use of estrogens and oral contraceptives induce reduction of vitamin B_6 level due to its excessive consumption. Diuretics and cortisone block the absorption of this vitamin [9, 20, 21]. Alcohol intake antagonizes vitamin B_6 status through production of acetaldehyde, which competes with PLP for binding sites of PLP-dependent enzymes [22].

Vitamin B_6 may itself act as an antagonist in patients with Parkinson's disease who are treated with L-dopa. In such cases, it can counteract the effect of L-dopa [23]. High doses of vitamin B_6 may lower blood concentrations of anticonvulsant medication such as phenytoin and phenobarbitone, apparently by increasing the rate of metabolism of the drugs [24].

Biological Activity

Vitamin B_6 is involved in more bodily functions than almost any other single nutrient. It affects both physical and mental health. Once digested, pyridoxine is converted rapidly to pyridoxal phosphate which acts as a co-enzyme in a whole host of biochemical reactions [25, 26]. Our interest will be concentrated on the nervous system in which it is required for normal brain function. Vitamin B_6 is involved in the synthesis of RNA and DNA, which contain the genetic instructions for the reproduction of all cells and for normal cellular growth.

It serves as a coenzyme of many enzymes involved in the metabolism of amino acids. Vitamin B_6 plays an important role in protein, carbohydrate and lipid metabolism. It helps in the transformation of amino acids to form active biogenic amines such as histamine, serotonin, dopamine, adrenaline and the formation of nicotinic acid. Furthermore, it removes an acid group from glutamic acid (glutamate) to form gamma-aminobutyric acid (GABA). Subsequent studies have found that GABA acts on the presynaptic nerve terminals to inhibit the release of excitatory neurotransmitters, thereby having a calming effect [27].

Toxicity

Vitamin B_6 is well tolerated in all its forms. Daily oral doses of pyridoxine of up to 50 times the RDA (approx. 100 mg) for periods up to 3–4 years have been administered without adverse effects. The lethal oral dose of pyridoxine, which kills 50% of rats, is 5500 mg/kg. The toxic dose of vitamin B_6 in dogs is known to be equivalent to 3,000 mg per day. Mega doses of pyridoxine will certainly cause toxic effects; there are reports that 1 gram per kg in rats may cause damage to peripheral nerves, degeneration of the spinal cord, and paralysis of the hind legs [8]. Fortunately, these side-effects are largely reversible upon cessation of vitamin B_6 intake. According to the US Government Institute of Medicine's Food and Nutrition Board, the minimum toxic dose of vitamin B_6 is 2,000 mg [28].

The development of sensory neuropathy has been described in patients who received 2–7 g/day of vitamin B_6 for a period of several months to two years [29, 30]. Other researchers have reported that 1–3 g/day of vitamin B_6 administered to healthy volunteers may lead to sensory neuropathy and progressive sensory ataxia. The symptoms continued to progress for 2–3 weeks after cessation of the supplements before regressing, even though PLP plasma concentrations had returned to normal [31]. There are polar opinions about the level of dose toxicity. Some researchers hold the idea that prolonged intake of doses exceeding 500 mg per day is considered to carry the risk of adverse side effects in certain persons, whereas 200 mg and less are believed to be safe [32-34]. On the opposite of these observations, it is important to note that both pyridoxine and PLP have been used quite extensively (intravenous PLP in doses of 40–50 mg/kg/d) for treatment of 574 children (aged 8 months to 15 years) with idiopathic epilepsy without obvious side-effects [35]. Bernard Rimland, who treated thousands of autistic children for long periods with high doses of vitamin B_6, stated that he has not seen any neurotoxic effects from this agent. He believes that such effects may result from deficiencies in magnesium and/or other nutrients which he prescribes in a balanced formula to complement the high levels of ingested vitamin B_6 [36]. Our experience with patients suffering from psychotropic drug-induced movement disorders, who were treated with high doses of vitamin B_6 (1,200 mg/day) from 5 days to 3 months, also did not demonstrate any neurological side effects during the studies, and continued using it over more than four years after ending the studies. Only one patient demonstrated acne during the vitamin phase, and another developed an allergic reaction (light itch) after a two-month treatment [37-40]. In the literature, few explanations can be found regarding the mechanism of development neurotoxicity induced by vitamin B_6. Rudman and Williams [41] have suggested mechanisms that may have caused this toxicity. In the first instance the dorsal root ganglia lie outside the blood brain barrier and are therefore not protected in the same way as the motor outflow from the spinal cord. Secondly, inactive circulating pyridoxine may occupy various enzyme sites and prevent access by the active pyridoxal-5-phosphate. It is interesting that Snell [42] had hypothesized many years previously that adverse reactions might result from accumulated pyridoxine for just this same reason.

Deficiency of Vitamin B_6

A dietary deficiency state showing definable clinical deficiency symptoms is rare, even though almost 50% of the diets evaluated in the 1977–78 US Food Consumption Study provided less than 70% of the recommended intake. Recent diet surveys revealed that a significant part of the population, especially elderly people, have B_6 intakes below the RDA. For that reason, people at risk of an insufficient pyridoxine status/intake are: pregnant and lactating women (this is due to the additional demands made by fetus or infant), women on oral contraceptive pills with a high estrogen content, chronic alcoholics (heavy drinking may severely impair the ability of the liver to synthesize PLP), and people with a high protein intake since protein metabolism depends upon the presence of pyridoxine [3, 9].

In cases of frank deficiency of a pyridoxine-depleted diet, it can lead to hypochromic anemia (abnormal decrease in the hemoglobin content of erythrocytes) and loss of ability to convert tryptophan to nicotinic acid. Antagonist-induced deficiency or certain genetic errors of amino acid metabolism may, if not duly treated, result in poor growth convulsions of cerebral origin, especially convulsive seizures in infants, decreased antibody formation, skin lesions (e.g., seborrheic dermatitis), abdominal distress, vomiting, kidney stones, electroencephalographic abnormalities, peripheral neuritis, and nerve degeneration [7, 9].

VITAMIN B_6 AND SCHIZOPHRENIA

Involvement of vitamin B_6 in organ function is extensive. Its deficiency can cause a broad spectrum of psychiatric symptoms. The mechanism of action is not yet clear enough, but many investigators have come to the conclusion that vitamin B_6 can be helpful in conditions such as autism [43-46], Alzheimer's disease [47], hyperactivity and learning disability [48], anxiety disorder [49, 50], premenstrual syndrome [51], schizophrenia [52, 53], and tardive dyskinesia [54-57]. In this chapter we will deal only with the application of this agent in psychotic disorders including schizophrenia, schizoaffective disorder, and the influence of psychotropic drugs on movement disturbances.

At the beginning of 1970s, few publications in the psychiatric literature raised concerns about pyridoxine's efficacy in treating schizophrenia [52, 53]. Since studies in those days were not methodically well built as controlled trials, and there was no systematic use of standard rating scales, the results were described mostly as clinical impression and not as monitored scientific data. As in many innovations in medicine, the first publications were of clinical case descriptions—for example, the case of a 15-year-old female presenting with psychotic symptoms secondary to homocysteinuria who responded to a combination of folic acid and pyridoxine [58]. Petrie and colleges found that pyridoxine has greater therapeutic effects in chronic schizophrenic patients [59]. Another case of "an unusual schizophrenic illness responsive to pyridoxine HCl (B_6) subsequent to phenothiazine and butyrophenone toxicities" was described in 1983 by Sidney Brooks and coworkers [53]. These authors reported on an 18-year-old male with schizophrenic symptoms who was successfully treated only with 500 mg/day of pyridoxine after a lot of somatic and neurological symptoms were induced by two different kinds of neuroleptic medications. Dose decreasing of vitamin B_6 led to deterioration of his mental symptoms, while returning to previous dose improved the patient's state back to the original balanced condition. In the next step, Bucci in 1970 started an open study in which he added 50 mg t.i.d. of pyridoxine to the treatment of 15 chronic schizophrenic patients without changing any other component of their treatment. The results were divided into a first period after 6 weeks when the positive effect was subjective only, but during the second period, after 8-10 weeks, the researcher had the impression of clinical improvement of affect, motivation and occupational ability [52].

Scanning the literature of the connection between vitamin B_6 and schizophrenia reveals two kinds of reports and studies. One direction examines the influence potential of the vitamin on basic symptoms, positive and negative, of the illness. The other direction seeks a resolution of various side effects induced by psychotropic drugs used for years before the days of the new generation drugs. In the upcoming part of this chapter, we would like to summarize the scientific information including our experience in this field.

As mentioned above, the problem with most previous studies and reports was the absence of control groups and the fact that data were based on general impression rather than on standard scientific tools [52, 53, 57, 59, 60].

Since vitamin B_6 is involved in the biosynthesis of the main neurotransmitters which are theoretically responsible for development of most psychiatric disorders, whether its baseline serum level is within the normal range was a basic and cardinal question.

It should be known that pyridoxine intake does not implicate its activity in body systems. The active form of pyridoxine is PLP, which is a derivative created by the enzyme pyridoxal kinase. In cases of an impaired pyridoxal kinase for the conversion of pyridoxine and pyridoxal to PLP, serum level of pyridoxine is between normal range or higher, while the PLP level will be very low. This was demonstrated in Adams and colleagues' study [61]. Therefore, in our recent vitamin B_6 studies we used the HPLC method which measures specific PLP levels [62].

We examined a group of "pure schizophrenic patients," i.e., those subjects who suffered only from core symptoms of the illness but not from any other disturbances such as movement disorders. This sample included 19 males and 30 females with a mean age of 49.2 ± 11.8 years (range 21–66 years). All patients were on a regular balanced hospital diet under the supervision of a clinical dietician, and there were no clinically relevant symptoms of malnutrition.

Blood samples (5 mL) were drawn before breakfast and first daily medication administration; it was immediately centrifuged for 10 min at room temperature and 3000 g, and the supernatant was frozen at –18°C until analyzed. All blood samples were drawn in light-proof test tubes and frozen serum also was kept in light-proof test tubes until analyzed. Measurement of the physiologically active vitamer of vitamin B_6 — PLP, was performed by HPLC separation according to Botticher and Botticher [62]. Plasma PLP concentration of more than 20 nmol/L was considered the normal level.

The results of this group's PLP levels were: total mean 26.3±13.5 nmol/L (range: 5.0–58.1); male 29.0±12.9 nmol/L (6.4–58.1); female 22.3±13.6 nmol/L (5–44). According to this finding we came to the conclusion that the "standard schizophrenic patient" has a normal PLP level. This finding has a special importance, since we have found a difference between schizophrenic and schizoaffective patients who have tardive dyskinesia (TD) as opposed to those who do not. We compared two groups: the first included 41 schizophrenic and schizoaffective patients with TD, and the control group included 49 schizophrenic subjects without TD. This comparison revealed a significantly lower level of PLP in the TD group especially among men: total mean was 17.7 ± 18.7 nmol/L (range 5.3–100.6 nmol/L); male 12.4±11.4 nmol/L (0–38.8); female 23.9±23.6 nmol/L (0–100.6).

Data presented above are taken from our last not-yet-published study (2006), but it contradicts our previous findings published in 2000 [17]. In that research, we did not find any difference between the TD group and the controls (45.4 ± 38.3 nmol/L and 39.0 ± 28.7 nmol/L, respectively). This contradiction can be explained by two components: 1) the new sample size was tripled, and 2) the use of different methods of vitamin B_6 measurement. In the last study, PLP was measured by the HPLC method as opposed to the previous study in which we used a radioenzymatic assay to detect pyridoxal. The HPLC method is characterized by direct measuring of all B_6 vitamers in plasma, in contrast to radioenzymatic assay, which allows detecting of all the vitamers together. The assessment of pyridoxal by radioenzymatic method is indirect, inaccurate, and its extrapolation is difficult [63].

VITAMIN B_6 AND PSYCHOTIC SYMPTOMS

As mentioned above, at the beginning of this part, some researchers had the clinical impression that vitamin B_6 has a beneficial effect on different mental conditions.

Use of vitamin B_6 in autism was pioneered by Bernard Rimland in the 1970s [36, 43]. Since then, thousands of children have been treated with doses ranging from 75–1,000 mg/day and without apparent serious side effects. The efficacy of B_6 in combination with magnesium has been demonstrated in properly controlled double-blind studies by Martineau et al. [64] and Lelord et al. [44] These studies have also demonstrated significant decreases in urinary homovanillic acid—one of the main dopamine metabolites. Carl Pfeiffer [65] has published a good deal over the years on the sub-typing of schizophrenia, including the concept of pyroluria—a condition which is supposedly responsive to vitamin B_6 and zinc. However, two years later, Cruz and Vogel [66] were unable to confirm pyroluria as a marker in chronic schizophrenia.

Recent studies have demonstrated that patients with schizophrenia often have elevated levels of homocysteine, which is suggested as a mediator of neurodeterioration or cognitive decline and negative symptoms in schizophrenia [67]. On the other hand, levels of vitamin B_6 and vitamin B_{12} are not different in schizophrenic patients compared to healthy subjects [68]. Levine et al. found that the addition of a B vitamin group (pyridoxine, folic acid and vitamin B_{12}) to ongoing antipsychotic treatment of schizophrenic patients led to significantly lower scores on the Positive and Negative Syndrome Scale (PANSS) in comparison with a placebo group [69].

There are some anecdotal reports (including ours) regarding the reduction of psychotic symptoms after vitamin B_6 supplementation in patients suffering from schizophrenia or organic mental disorder [52, 57, 60, 70, 71], but only three studies were performed on comparatively large groups of patients. Unfortunately, these were not controlled studies, and no conclusive clinical trials have yet been undertaken [52, 70, 71]. We thus decided to examine whether vitamin B_6 influences psychotic symptoms in patients suffering from refractory schizophrenia and schizoaffective disorder, using a double-blind, crossover, add-on design study [72].

About six years ago we performed a study regarding vitamin B_6 as a treatment of tardive dyskinesia [73]. As a by-product of this study, we examined the influence of vitamin B_6 on the patients' positive symptoms [72]. It must be highlighted that the doses of pyridoxine were relatively low (maximum 400 mg/day), while the patients were severely chronic and treatment resistant.

Even though our sample contained the most severe chronic patients, the results of this study showed an improvement in various degrees in five of 15 patients (30%). However, these results were not considered positive because only two of the five patients demonstrated significant clinical improvement. In two recent studies regarding high doses (1,200mg/day) of vitamin B_6 as a treatment of acute akathisia, we examined again its influence on positive symptoms [38, 39]. In these double-blind randomized control studies, the patients suffered from acute schizophrenic exacerbation and were not chronic or treatment resistant. The results clearly demonstrated a significant reduction of positive signs in BPRS compared to those patients on placebo.

VITAMIN B_6 AND COGNITION

Micronutrient status can affect cognitive function at all ages. Vitamin deficiencies could influence memory function and might contribute to age-associated cognitive impairment and dementia. Results of experimental animal models studies suggest that serious cognitive deficit may occur also in vitamin B_6-deficient animals [74, 75]. The authors suggest that vitamin B_6 deficiency during gestation and lactation alters the function of N-methyl-D-aspartate receptors, which play an important role in learning and memory. Low levels of vitamin B_6 due to poor dietary intake are not uncommon in the elderly and have been related to cognitive decline and memory dysfunction. However, the underlying mechanism is not known. Studies have suggested the effect of vitamin B_6 on cognition may be mediated by vascular white matter lesions, given evidence that low vitamin B_6 levels may result in premature vascular disease, possibly due to high levels of homocysteine. Recently Mulder and colleagues found a linear relationship between white matter lesions and hippocampal atrophy in patients with probable Alzheimer's disease, suggesting that vascular pathology and typical Alzheimer's disease pathology are related [76, 77].

Numerous studies have suggested that pregnant and lactating women may have dietary intake of vitamin B_6 that are well below the recommended dietary allowance, which may affect the vitamin B_6 status of their offspring [75].

A few recent studies have demonstrated an association between declines in cognitive function or Alzheimer's disease in the elderly and inadequate nutritional status of folic acid, vitamin B_{12}, and vitamin B_6 and thus, elevated levels of homocysteine [78]. One observational study found higher plasma vitamin B_6 levels to be associated with better performance on two measures of memory, but unrelated to performance on 18 other cognitive tests [79]. It is presently unclear whether marginal B vitamin deficiencies, which are relatively common in the elderly, contribute to age-associated declines in cognitive function or whether both result from processes associated with aging and/or disease. Malouf et al. mentioned in their review that there are no evidence found for short-term benefit from vitamin B_6 in improving mood (depression, fatigue and tension symptoms) or cognitive functions [77]. They come to the conclusion that more randomized controlled trials are needed to explore possible benefits from vitamin B_6 supplementation for healthy older people and those with cognitively impairment or dementia.

VITAMIN B_6 AND PSYCHOTROPIC-INDUCED MOVEMENT DISORDERS

Abnormalities of serotonin (5-HT) metabolism have been associated with various neurological conditions including Parkinson's disease, tardive dyskinesia, akathisia, dystonia, Huntington's disease, familial tremor, restless leg syndrome, myoclonus, Gilles de la Tourette syndrome, multiple sclerosis, sleep disorders and dementia. The natural precursor of serotonin, L-tryptophan is hydroxylated by tryptophan hydroxylase to L-5-hydroxytryptophan (L-5HTP) and then it is decarboxylated to serotonin by pyridoxal phosphate-dependent enzyme – vitamin B_6 and aromatic amino acid decarboxylases [80].

Although there are descriptions of many movement disorders that can be connected to vitamin B_6 deficiency, we would like to deal in this chapter only with those movement disturbances induced by psychotropic drugs. This group of motor disorders includes acute akathisia, lithium-induced tremor and tardive dyskinesia (TD). It is well known that most acute movement disturbances of extrapyramidal origin may be successfully treated by the use of anticholinergic agents and other drugs.

Acute Akathisia

The condition of an "inability to be seated" was described by Haskovec more than 100 years ago [81]. Now termed akathisia, it is used exclusively for a description of neuroleptic-drug-induced irritability. Although the use of novel antipsychotic agents has led to fewer patients developing drug-induced movement disorders, acute akathisia remains a common finding among psychiatric patients treated by both conventional and atypical neuroleptics. Usually acute akathisia develops within a few days to weeks of initiating or raising the dose of neuroleptic medications or after reducing dosages of medications used to treat extrapyramidal symptoms [82]. According to DSM-IV criteria, the condition describes subjective complaints of restlessness accompanied by observed movements such as fidgeting of the legs, rocking from foot to foot, pacing, or an inability to sit or stand still. Incidence rates for acute akathisia with conventional neuroleptics vary from 8% to 76%, with 20% to 30% being a conservative estimate [83]. Although the atypical antipsychotics represent a great advance in terms of their tolerability profiles, they are still associated with some risk of acute akathisia, with described incidence rates of up to 18% among patients treated by atypicals alone [84].

Early intervention when drug-induced akathisia appears usually leads to better patient confidence and compliance with subsequent neuroleptic therapy. The pathogenesis of akathisia remains unclear, with various theories suggested. It is suggested that an imbalance of several neurotransmitter systems (such as dopamine, norepinephrine, acetylcholine, gamma aminobutyric acid [GABA], and serotonin) in tegmental and nigrostriatal areas may be involved in the pathogenetic process [85, 86]. We have previously suggested that free radicals may be involved in the pathogenesis [38]. Treatment strategies against acute neuroleptic-induced akathisia include anticholinergic (antimuscarinic) agents, dopamine agonists, GABA-ergic agents, beta-blockers, benzodiazepines and serotonin antagonists. However, many patients suffering from acute akathisia fail to respond.

In the process of researching the efficacy of vitamin B_6 as a treatment for acute neuroleptic-induced akathisia (NIA), we performed two double-blind studies [38, 39]. In the first we compared the effect of vitamin B_6 vs. placebo [38].

The study was conducted in two mental health centers. Inclusion criteria for this study were a) DSM-IV criteria for acute NIA; b) a score of at least two (mild akathisia) on the global subscale of the Barnes Akathisia Scale (BARS) [87]; c) the doses of all medications were to remain unchanged for at least three days before the baseline ratings and during the entire study period of five days; and d) all patients had to be hospitalized. Patients were not included if anticholinergic agents were started less than 10 days before screening. Furthermore, patients receiving beta-adrenergic receptor antagonists and/or vitamin therapy were excluded.

Twenty inpatients (14 men and six women) were enrolled in the study. Their ages ranged from 21 to 69 years old (mean 42.4 years, SD = 14.7). All patients received neuroleptic agents. Fourteen patients received conventional psychotropic drugs (chlorpromazine equivalent 300–900 mg/day, mean 438±195.2 mg/day). Six (equal in both vitamin and placebo groups) received atypical antipsychotics (three patients risperidone 4–8 mg/day, mean 6±2 mg/day, and three olanzapine 1,020 mg/day, mean 16.6±5.8 mg/day). Eleven patients (six in the vitamin B_6 group and five in the placebo group) were treated with combination therapy (antipsychotic and valproic acid (800–2,000 mg/day, mean 1314.3±429.8 mg/day) or lithium (800–1,200 mg/day, mean 1350±173.2 mg/day). Treatment with an anticholinergic agent (trihexyphenidyl)—which had begun prior to the appearance of NIA—to treat parkinsonian symptoms, was continued in eight patients (four in the vitamin B_6 group and four in the placebo group), at doses ranging between 2–6 mg/day (mean 4.2±1.28 mg/day). In these patients, NIA appeared and persisted in spite of this treatment. The average time of unchanged dose medications before the study beginning was 12.3±4.2 days.

The diagnosis of NIA was established by clinical interview. All the patients developed akathisia after just a few days from the exposure to a new neuroleptic drug. There was no relationship between the akathisia and psychotic irritability. Furthermore, the patients complained of a sense of being driven and an awareness of tension and discomfort in the lower limbs, which is one of the distinguishing criteria between akathisia and psychotic agitation [87-89]. The severity of akathisia was rated by the Barnes Akathisia Rating Scale (BARS) [87] on baseline and every day during the study. All patients were assessed by the same investigators followed by a pretrial training period. Inasmuch as the study was done in two mental centers, interrater reliability of raters on the BARS was examined: the kappa was 0.89. Clinically relevant response was defined as a reduction of at least two points on the BARS global subscale. All assessments were made in the morning at the same time of day (8:00 AM ± 1:00 hour), before drug administration. All participants were physically healthy, and the results of routine laboratory tests were within normal range.

The study design was double-blind placebo-controlled. Twenty selected inpatients for this study were randomly divided to receive either vitamin B_6 1,200mg/day (n=10) or placebo (n=10) twice a day for five days. Clinical and demographic characteristics are presented in Table 2.

All patients completed the trial. None of them suffered from any side effect. Since there is a significant difference between vitamin B_6 and placebo groups regarding age ($p < .05$) (Table 2), we performed repeated ANCOVA measures with the age as covariate and gender and time as grouping factors. This analysis showed no significant interaction between gender, time, and age ($F= 0.50$; df 5, 90; $P = 0.77$). The mean baseline rating for the BARS subscales also were similar. The mean changes from baseline in each of the BARS subscale scores are presented in Table 3. A significant difference between baseline and final rating in all scales was demonstrated. Ratings of objective subscale showed a trend of improvement in the vitamin B_6 group, but it did not approach a significant level ($P <.079$). The subjective subscale (awareness of restlessness and distress related to restlessness) and global clinical assessment subscales showed a significant two-way interaction of treatment and time. Vitamin B_6 produced a greater improvement in NIA than in patients from the placebo group. This beneficial effect was revealed from the third day. The same effect was obtained in the global subscale from the second day.

Table 2. Demographic, Clinical Characteristics and Baseline Rating Scale Score in Vitamin B_6 and Placebo Groups with Acute Neuroleptic-Induced Akathisia

Variables	Vitamin B_6	Placebo	P
Age (years)	36.2 (14.6)	48.7 (12.4)	=0.0538
Gender (male : female)	9:1	5:5	=0.1432*
Duration of illness (years)	13.0 (21.2)	8.23 (14.7)	NS
Duration of akathisia (days)			
Mean	11.1 (9.5)	8.1 (14.9)	NS
Range	4–23	2–27	
Diagnosis			
Schizophrenia	6	5	
Schizoaffective disorders	4	4	NS
Mood disorders	-	1	
Treatment:			
Atypical antipsychotics	3	3	NS
Antipsychotics + Valproate or Lithium	6	5	NS
Antiparkinsonian drugs	4	4	NS
Baseline scores			
BPRS	50.2 (8.3)	47.5 (7.8)	NS
CGI	4.7 (0.48)	4.6 (0.51)	NS
BARS:			
Objective subscale	2.7 (0.48)	2.5 (0.52)	NS
Subjective subscales:			
Awareness of restlessness	2.7 (0.48)	2.4 (0.51)	NS
Distress related to restlessness	2.5 (0.52)	2.3 (0.48)	NS
Global subscale	4.1 (0.73)	3.8 (0.78)	NS

BPRS – Brief Psychiatric Rating Scale; CGI – Clinical Global Assessments;
BARS – Barnes Akathisia Rating Scale.
*Yates corrected $\chi 2$.

As some of the patients were treated only with antipsychotics and others with a combination of antipsychotics and mood stabilizers (valproate and lithium), we compared these groups in order to examine whether an influence of the different treatments on the improvement of akathisia exists. It did not reveal any significant difference between the groups ($P>.12$). We can suggest that vitamin B_6 ameliorated the akathisia signs but not the neuroleptic-induced dysphoria.

Furthermore, according to the definition of response as a reduction of at least two points on the BARS global assessment subscale, the number of responders is significantly greater in the vitamin B_6 group (8/10, 80%), than in the placebo group (3/10, 30%) ($P=.037$). A complete disappearance of NIA (BARS global score = 0) occurred in three patients (30.0%) in the vitamin B_6 group and in one in the placebo group (10.0%). Only two patients in the vitamin group showed insignificant clinical improvement on this scale (one point on this subscale), whereas in the placebo group there were six such patients and the state of one patient remained without any changes. The results of this study showed that the treatment of patients suffering from acute akathisia with vitamin B_6 led to improvement of NIA symptoms within a few days [38].

Table 3. Effect of Vitamin B_6 and Placebo in Patients with Acute Neuroleptic-Induced Akathisia (results are expressed as mean (SD))

BARS subscale	Groups	Baseline	Day 1	Day 2	Day 3	Day 4	Day 5	F*	d.f.	P
Objective	Vitamin	2.7 (0.48)	1.7 (0.67)	1.4 (0.96)	1.2 (0.79)	1.4 (1.26)	0.8 (0.92)	2.04	5, 90	=0.0797
	Placebo	2.5 (0.52)	2.3 (0.48)	1.9 (0.57)	1.8 (0.79)	1.6 (0.97)	1.7 (0.82)			
Subjective awareness of restlessness	Vitamin	2/7 (0.48)	1.9 (0.87)	1.1 (0.87)	1.0 (1.05)	1.2 (1.13)	0.7 (0.82)	5.07	5, 90	=0.0004
	Placebo	2.4 (0.51)	2.2 (0.42)	2.1 (0.57)	2.2 (0.63)	1.9 (0.87)	2.0 (0.94)			
Distress related to restlessness	Vitamin	2.5 (0.53)	1.7 (0.82)	0.9 (1.10)	0.7 (0.82)	0.8 (1.13)	0.6 (0.84)	3.2	5, 90	=0.0105
	Placebo	2.3 (0.48)	2.1 (0.31)	1.6 (0.70)	1.8 (0.91)	1.3 (1.05)	1.6 (0.84)			
Global	Vitamin	4.1 (0.74)	2.8 (0.92)	2.2 (1.23)	1.7 (0.95)	1.6 (1.17)	1.2 (1.13)	3.74	5, 90	=0.0040
	Placebo	3.8 (0.79)	3.4 (0.97)	3.0 (0.94)	2.9 (1.10)	2.3 (1.25)	2.6 (1.34)			

BARS – Barnes Akathisia Rating Scale.

Table 4. Effect of Vitamin B_6, Mianserin and Placebo in Patients with Acute Neuroleptic-Induced Akathisia (results are expressed as mean (SD))

BARS subscale	Groups	Baseline	Day 1	Day 2	Day 3	Day 4	Day 5	F*	d.f.	P
Objective	Vitamin	2.5 (0.6)	1.9 (0.8)	1.7 (1.0)	1.5 (0.9)	1.4 (1.0)	1.4 (0.9)	1.8227	10, 285	=.05643
	Mianserin	2.6 (0.6)	2.1(0.8)	1.8(0.8)	1.7(0.8)	1.5 (1.0)	1.4(1.0)			
	Placebo	2.4 (0.5)	2.3(0.5)	2.0(0.4)	2.2(0.5)	2.2(0.4)	2.2(0.4)			
Subjective awareness of restlessness	Vitamin	2.7 (0.5)	2.1(0.9)	1.4(1.0)	1.2(1.0)	1.2(1.0)	1.0(1.0)	6.734	10, 285	<.0001
	Mianserin	2.7 (0. 6)	2.2(0.8)	1.8(0.8)	1.5(0.7)	1.4(0.8)	1.2(0.9)			
	Placebo	2.4 (0.6)	2.2(0.5)	1.9(0.7)	2.4(0.6)	2.2(0.4)	2.4(0.5)			
Distress related to restlessness	Vitamin	2.5 (0.6)	1.9(0.9)	1.3(1.0)	1.0(0.92)	1.0(1.0)	0.9(0.9)	6.9460	10, 285	<.0001
	Mianserin	2.4 (0.7)	1.9(0.8)	1.6(0.8)	1.4(0.9)	1.3(0.9)	1.1(1.0)			
	Placebo	2.4 (0.5)	2.2(0.4)	1.9(0.4)	2.3(0.6)	2.2(0.4)	2.4(0.5)			
Global	Vitamin	3.9 (0.9)	3.0(1.1)	2.4(1.2)	2.2(1.1)	1.9(1.3)	1.7(1.3)	6.243	10, 285	<.0001
	Mianserin	3.7 (1.0)	3.1(1.0)	2.7(0.9)	2.0(0.9)	1.9(1.1)	1.5(1.1)			
	Placebo	3.6 (0.7)	3.4(0.8)	3.1(0.9)	3.1(0.8)	3.1(0.7)	3.3(0.9)			

* - ANOVA/MANOVA two-way interaction.

In spite of the encouraging results reported for 5-HT_{2a} antagonists, these agents fail to yield a response in a substantial proportion of NIA patients. Furthermore, some studies of atypical novel antipsychotics have found that despite their high 5-HT_{2a} receptor occupancy rate (> 90%), they may still induce EPS and akathisia [86]. This suggests that the protective action of 5-HT_{2a} blockers against akathisia due to D_2 blockade may not be universal, and that other pathophysiological mechanisms may be involved [90].

Some open [91, 92] and double-blind studies [93] have demonstrated the effectiveness of mianserin (15mg/day) in the treatment of patients with acute NIA. In the next step, we compared the efficacy of vitamin B_6 versus mianserin and placebo as an add-on treatment of NIA [39].

Mianserin is a tetracyclic antidepressant with marked 5-HT_{2a} and 5-HT_{2c} antagonism as well as antihistaminergic and α-2 antagonistic activity, without anticholinergic properties. The results of studies evaluating serotonin-active agents with predominant affinity for different subtypes of 5-HT receptors indicate that within the 5-HT system, the 5-HT_{2a} receptors are those that are involved in the pharmacotherapy of acute NIA [86, 94-96].

This double-blind placebo-controlled study was conducted in the same two mental health centers, with the same inclusion and exclusion criteria. Of 67 screened subjects, 60 inpatients (35 men and 25 women) suffering from schizophrenia (35 patients), schizoaffective disorder (25 patients) and bipolar affective disorder (five patients) were enrolled in the study. All patients were in an acute phase of their illness. There was no relationship between the akathisia and psychotic irritability. All inpatients eligible for this study were randomly assigned to receive either vitamin B_6 1,200mg/day (n=23) or mianserin 15 mg/day (n=20), or placebo (n=17) twice daily for five days.

All patients successfully completed the study with none suffering adverse events. There were no significant differences between patients in each group according to sex, age, diagnosis, duration of illness and akathisia and their previous treatment. The mean baseline rating for the BARS subscales did not differ between the groups (Table 4). A significant difference between baseline and final rating in all scales was demonstrated in both treatment groups, but not in the placebo group. Ratings on the objective subscale showed a trend towards improvement in the mianserin and vitamin B_6 group, but did not approach significance (P>.05). The subjective subscale (awareness of restlessness and distress related to restlessness) and global clinical assessment subscale showed a significant two-way interaction of treatment and time. Vitamin B_6 and mianserin produced a greater improvement in NIA than in patients receiving a placebo. This beneficial effect was revealed from the third day in the vitamin group, and from the fifth day in the mianserin group, respectively. Vitamin B_6 and mianserin also led to improvement of NIA on the distress subscale from the third and fourth day, respectively. The same effect was obtained in the global subscale from the fifth day in both treatment groups.

Complete disappearance of the NIA occurred in 22% of patients in the vitamin B_6 group and in 20% of patients in the mianserin group, but in none of the patients in the placebo group.

The efficacy of vitamin B_6 suggests that the pathophysiology of acute NIA is heterogeneous with various subtypes of acute NIA, which possibly respond to different pharmacologic approaches. Our results suggest that vitamin B_6 also may be an option in the treatment of acute akathisia.

Vitamin B_6 and Lithium-induced Tremor

The beneficial effect on parkinsonian signs in our previous studies encouraged us to investigate the possible effect of vitamin B_6 on drug-induced movement disorder of drugs other than neuroleptics. Lithium is such a drug and "lithium-induced tremor" (LT) is one of its most common adverse effects. Tremor is a general term that defines a regular continuous and rhythmical involuntary oscillation of a body part [97].

Five outpatients who were treated only with ligium were suffering from. In addition to their medication regimen, they received oral vitamin B_6 (900–1,200 mg per day). According to the Simpson-Angus Scale (SAS) scores, four patients showed an impressive improvement until total disappearance of the tremor. Only one patient did not have any improvement. The subjective scale, in which the patients scored their impression of clinical improvement, showed similar results. One patient reported total recovery, another three patients reported marked improvement and only one patient did not feel any change. None of the patients suffered from any side effects attributable to vitamin B_6. At the end of the study three patients discontinued the vitamin B_6 treatment with recurrence of the tremor to previous levels. In these patients we recommenced treatment with vitamin B_6 and the same beneficial effect was achieved. A follow-up of ten months did not reveal any side effects and the therapeutic effect was maintained [37].

Our preliminary results on the use of vitamin B_6 in lithium-induced tremor suggest that it may be an efficacious therapy. The mechanism of the tremor caused by lithium is still unclear and so is the mechanism of its amelioration by vitamin B_6 treatment. However, there is a trial of explanation by some authors. Kane et al. [98] reported that 38 patients treated only with lithium had developed parkinsonian symptoms. Tyrer et al. explained the appearance of extrapyramidal side effects after treatment with lithium by selective blockade of dopamine receptors [99, 100]. These reports can be a clue suggesting the connection between lithium or neuroleptic-induced tremor and vitamin B_6.

Vitamin B_6 and Tardive Dyskinesia

Tardive dyskinesia (TD) is a common adverse effect generally caused by chronic use of classic neuroleptics. The long-term delayed neurological side effects of these drugs are determined as tardive movement disorders. This term contains some variable types: classical TD, and other tardive extrapyramidal subsyndromes [101–109]. The prevalence of TD among subjects treated with classic neuroleptics over more than one year ranges from 3% to as high as 70% (depending on the diagnostic criteria and/or methodology) [105, 110, 111]. The annual incidence in younger adults is 4% to 5% [111, 112]. Many cases are persistent, often irreversible, and may result in social and physiological impairment.

Although second generation agents (SGAs) have a significant reduction potential for causing acute and tardive neuroleptic-induced extrapyramidal symptoms including TD [113–115], each of them may also induce tardive movement disturbances [116–125]. Furthermore, despite the extensive use of SGAs in the majority of western countries, most patients in countries of the third world and up to half in Europe are still treated with classic neuroleptics.

A large number of different medications have been studied in the treatment of TD patients, but its management remains a significant problem for patients, and a therapeutic riddle for physicians [126].

Some researchers reported on motor disturbances which have been observed in vitamin B_6-deficient animals [127, 128]. Preliminary evidence in humans demonstrates efficacy of vitamin B_6 in treatment of TD and other involuntary drug-induced movement disorders published as several case reports [54–57, 60, 129], open-label trials [37, 130], and randomized, double-blind, placebo-controlled trials [38–40, 73].

In our previous report, in open and double-blind studies [60, 73, 130], we evaluated the efficacy of vitamin B_6 in treatment of TD with relatively small doses (up to 400mg/day) and found it effective. Our clinical experience with this compound showed a positive effect of vitamin B_6 on TD connected to its dose, an effect that continued for a long period after stopping the high dose of the medication (1,200 mg/day).

The subjects were all inpatients who fulfilled the following inclusion criteria: a) DSM-IV diagnosis of schizophrenia or schizoaffective disorder; b) a diagnosis of TD (according to DSM-IV-TR research criteria [131]) confirmed independently by three specialized psychiatrists well-experienced in the diagnosis and treatment of movement disorders; c) moderate severity of each of the psychotropic drug-induced movement, as measured by the clinical global impression of severity of the Extrapyramidal Symptom Rating Scale (ESRS) [132, 133]; d) signs and symptoms of TD developed either during exposure to a neuroleptic medication, or within four weeks of withdrawal from oral neuroleptics or within eight weeks of withdrawal from a depot form; e) exposure to psychotropic medication for at least three months prior to the appearance of the movement disorders; f) duration of symptoms for at least one year; and g) a stable psychotropic regimen over at least one month prior to entry into the study.

All patients were on a regular balanced hospital diet under the supervision of a clinical dietician, and there were no clinically relevant symptoms of malnutrition.

Fifty patients (28 men and 22 women) were enrolled into the study. The mean ± SD age was 47±11 years (range 20–66 years). Thirty-four patients suffered from chronic schizophrenia and 16 patients from schizoaffective disorder. All patients had been hospitalized for one to three years. Most of them were smokers and suffered from TD and other extrapyramidal symptoms less than five years. The patients' characteristics are presented in Table 5.

The psychotropic medication regimen remained unchanged throughout the study. Thirty-two patients received conventional (the average dose of current antipsychotic medications was 396.7 ± 280.4 mg/day in chlorpromazine equivalent), and 19 patients received atypical antipsychotics.

After baseline assessment, the subjects were randomly assigned to receive, under double-blind conditions, either tablets of vitamin B_6, or an appearance- and taste-matched placebo, for 26 weeks. Each patient received either vitamin B_6 twice a day (1,200mg/day) or placebo twice a day. After a two-week washout period (following vitamin or placebo treatment), the patients received the next 12 weeks of treatment with the other preparation. Vitamin B_6 or placebo were given in addition to each patient's regular antipsychotic medication. Both patients and physicians were blinded to group allocation. A crossover design was used as an appropriate design for chronic patients in stable pathologic condition, in an attempt to reduce variance and increase effective sample size.

Table 5. Demographic Data and Clinic Characteristic of Patients Suffering from Tardive Dyskinesia

	Whole sample (N=50)	Randomization Vitamin B_6 (N=28)	Placebo (N=22)
Gender (N):			
Female	22	12	10
Male	28	16	12
Age (years):			
Mean:	46.8±11.1	45.4±12.3	48.5±9.4
Range:	20–66	20–62	29–66
Smokers	46	26	20
Nonsmokers	4	2	2
DSM-IV diagnosis:			
Schizophrenia	34	18	16
Schizoaffective Disorder	16	10	6
Duration of illness (years):			
Mean:	19.0±10.9	18.6±10.0	19.5±9.2
Range:	2–41	2–41	4–34
Duration of TD (years):			
<3	28	16 (57%)	12 (54%)
3–5	10	5 (18%)	5 (23%)
>5	12	7 (25%)	5 (23%)
Treatment (N):			
Typical antipsychotics	32	17(61%)	15 (68%)
Atypical antipsychotics	19	10 (36%)	9 (41%)
Mood stabilizers	18	11 (39%)	7 (32%)

Results are expressed as mean and SD.

Severity of movement disorders was assessed by the ESRS, an experimental tool that was developed by G. Chouinard and A. Ross-Chouinard for epidemiological studies of tardive dyskinesia in schizophrenic patients chronically treated with various antipsychotic agents. It was also designed to rate four types of drug-induced movement disorders (both acute and delayed-onset [tardive]): parkinsonism, akathisia, dystonia and tardive dyskinesia. Its sensitivity and validity was established through several clinical trials [132, 133]. The parkinsonism subscale includes the assessment of proper parkinsonian symptoms (expressive automatic movements, bradykinesia, rigidity, gait and posture, sialorrhea and postural stability), as well as the assessment of tremor and akathisia. In addition, ESRS also includes a clinical global impression subscale (CGI).

Safety and tolerability of high doses of vitamin B_6 were evaluated by assessing the incidence and severity of adverse events for each phase of the study for all patients who had received at least one dose of study medication during that phase, as well as withdrawals because of adverse events.

Table 6. Efficacy of Vitamin B_6 vs. Placebo in Schizophrenic Patients with Tardive Movement Disorders in Period 1 (ESRS subscales analysis, mean ±SEM, n=45)

ESRS subscales	Treatment	Baseline†	Time				Treatment effect (df = 1, 43)	Time (df = 4, 172)	Time-Treatment interaction (df = 4, 172)
			Week 2	Week 4	Week 8	Week 12			
Tardive Parkinsonism	Vitamin N=23	28.3±2.1	18.0±2.5	14.1±2.4	11.6±2.1	9.8±2.0*	F=10.7; p<.002	F=24.6; p<.00001	F=13.1; p<.00001
	Placebo N=22	26.8±2.2	25.5±2.6	24.4±2.4	23.9±2.2	25.4±2.1			
Tardive Dyskinesia	Vitamin N=23	9.9±1.5	7.6±1.3	6.4±1.1	5.3±1.2	4.7±0.9	F=0.09; p=.760	F=3.6; p<.0002	F=6.3; p<.00009
	Placebo N=22	6.6±1.5	7.4±1.2	7.7±1.3	7.2±1.4	7.4±1.3			
Clinical Global Impression	Vitamin N=23	4.3±0.2	3.5±0.2	3.0±0.2	2.3±0.2*	1.9±0.2**	F=13.3; p<.0001	F=29.5; p<.0001	F=20.1; p<.0001
	Placebo N=22	4.1±0.2	4.0±0.2	4.0±0.2	3.9±0.3	3.9±0.2			

† - No difference between groups baseline p>.05
* - LSD Post Hoc Test p<.025
** - LSD Post Hoc Test p<.01
ESRS – Extrapyramidal Symptom Rating Scale
SEM – Standard Error

Table 7. Efficacy of Vitamin B_6 vs. Placebo in Schizophrenic Patients with Tardive Movement Disorders (ESRS subscales analysis, mean ±SEM, n=36)

ESRS subscales	Treatment	Baseline†	Improvement (Δ from baseline)				Treatment effect (df = 1, 34)	Treatment x Time (df = 3, 102)	Treatment x time x order interaction (df = 3, 102)*
Tardive Parkinsonism	Vitamin	24.1±1.8	5.6±0.9	10.3±1.2**	12.6±1.3**	14.9±1.5**	F=45.3; p<.00001	F=25.0; p<.00001	F=2.3; p<.09
Tardive Dyskinesia	Vitamin	8.7±1.1	1.4±0.5	2.7±0.7	3.8±0.9*	4.2±0.8*	F=17.9; p<.0001	F=8.7; p<.0003	F=2.2; p<.09
Clinical Global Impression	Vitamin	4.0±0.1	0.7±0.1	1.2±0.2*	1.7±0.2**	2.0±0.2**	F=60.6; p<.0001	F=26.5; p<.0001	F=6.2; p<.0001

† - No difference between groups baseline p>.05
* - LSD Post Hoc Test p<.01
** - LSD Post Hoc Test p<.005
ESRS – Extrapyramidal Symptom Rating Scale
SEM – Standard Error

All patients were assessed by the same investigators, who had undergone pretrial training in the assessment tool. The assessment was performed at baseline, weeks 2, 4, 8, 12 (end of period I), on the 14th week (end of washout period), and on weeks 16, 18, 22, 26 (end of period II). All study and routine medications were taken by the participants in the presence of nursing staff. This careful monitoring ensured compliance.

A 20% reduction in ESRS scores from baseline to week 12 on the rating scales was taken to represent no response; 21–40% as minimal improvement; 41–60% as moderate improvement and more than 61% as marked improvement [73].

Most patients tolerated vitamin B_6 well, and were able to receive the maximal dose of 1,200 mg/day during the whole study. Only one patient demonstrated acne during the vitamin phase and another developed an allergic reaction (light itch) after a two-month treatment. Forty-five subjects completed the first phase, and 36 both phases of the study.

Three-way repeated measures of the ANOVA for the two-period crossover design revealed significant differences between vitamin B6 and placebo groups in scores on the dyskinetic movement subscale in phase 1 and phase 2. Figures 5, 6, and 7 illustrate ESRS scores during the two-period crossover design treatment. Table 6 demonstrates efficacy of vitamin B_6 vs. placebo during phase 1. Table 7 shows the changes of ESRS (parkinsonism, dyskinetic subscales, and CGI) from baseline to endpoint including the checking stations.

Among the 45 patients (23 on vitamin B_6 and 22 on placebo) who completed the first phase of the study, 21 patients (91%) of those who were treated with vitamin B_6 demonstrated different levels of clinical improvement: eight (35%) patients showed marked, seven (30%) patients moderate, and six (26%) patients showed minimal improvement. Only two (9%) patients remained without any change. Among 22 patients who were treated with placebo, three (14%) patients demonstrated minimal improvement. Seventeen patients (77 %) did not show any effect and the condition became worse in two (9%) patients ($\chi^2 = 29.7$, df=3, $P < .0001$).

The analysis of the baseline scores of parkinsonism, dyskinetic movements and CGI subscales of these 45 patients, did not reveal any significant difference between the vitamin and placebo groups (Table 7).

A highly significant therapeutic effect of vitamin B_6 in the parkinsonism, dyskinetic and CGI subscales was found. The parkinsonism scores diminished from baseline (28.3) to endpoint (9.8) during vitamin B_6 treatment a total of 18.5 points, and only 1.4 points (from 26.8 to 25.4) during placebo treatment, p=.00001. Significant improvement in parkinsonism subscale appeared in the 12th week of treatment with vitamin B_6, $p<.01$. Symptoms of tardive dyskinesia diminished 5.2 points from baseline (9.9) to the endpoint (4.7) in patients treated with vitamin B_6, in contrast to patients who received placebo whose scores increased 0.8 points (from 6.6 to 7.4 points, p=.00009). The CGI rates diminished 2.4 points (from 4.3 to 1.9) and almost were not changed with placebo—4.1 at baseline and 3.9 at endpoint, $p<.0001$. Improvement was significant from the 8th week, $p<.01$ (Table 7).

In contrast to phase 1, in which the baseline scores of both groups were identical, in phase 2 the starting scores were different due to the influence of the carryover effect of previous vitamin therapy (Table 5, Table 6, and Table 7). Changes in clinical impression and ESRS scores showed that vitamin B_6 was significantly more effective than placebo: symptoms of tardive parkinsonism decreased by 14.9±1.5 units from baseline to endpoint, and -4.9±1.8 units with placebo, $p<.00001$; dyskinetic symptoms were diminished from baseline to endpoint for a total of 4.2±0.8 units during vitamin treatment, and -2.9±0.9 during placebo, $p<.0003$; CGI rates changed 2.0 ± 0.2 during vitamin treatment in contrast to -0.6 ± 0.2 with placebo, $p<.00001$. A significant difference in the parkinsonism subscale demonstrated improvement starting the fourth week of vitamin B_6 treatment, $p<.004$; in the dyskinetic subscale a significant improvement appeared from the 8th week of treatment with vitamin B_6, $p<.01$). The CGI subscale showed a significant positive effect from the 4th week of vitamin B_6 treatment, $p<.004$ (Table 7).

Continuous beneficial effect of vitamin B_6 was observed in all ESRS subscales, but the most prominent impressive significance was demonstrated in the CGI subscale (Table 6). After two weeks of washout period, the patients with placebo substitution in the second phase showed no significant difference in CGI rates until the fourth week. Right after this period of time the CGI score demonstrated returning to pre-vitamin treatment state and at the 12th week they came back almost to baseline level of ESRS scores.

The results of this double-blind placebo-controlled study suggest that a high dose of vitamin B_6 (1,200 mg/day) is an effective and safe treatment for TD and other extrapyramidal symptoms. A positive effect was seen not only during the treatment period, but continuing for approximately eight weeks after stopping it. The high-dose vitamin B_6 acts for a longer period in comparison to lower doses (400 mg/day), which were also found to be effective but not for longer than one week after discontinuing the treatment, according to our previous double-blind study [73].

Conclusions

In conventional medicine and psychiatry up to the present date there is not enough understanding about the causes of mental diseases, and the commonly-used treatments, such as antipsychotics, antidepressants and other psychotropic drugs (such as sedatives and stimulants), and electroconvulsive therapy and psychotherapy, address symptoms only and do not always lead to termination of the psychiatric problem.

Natural medicine and food supplement use offer additional insight into these conditions. Normal mental functioning needs an optimal presence of biogenic amines such as dopamine, serotonin, norepinephrine, acetylcholine and others. Vitamin B_6 or pyridoxine is essential for the metabolism and synthesis of proteins, including all of the neurotransmitters mentioned above. Vitamin B_6 deficiency can cause many psychiatric and somatic disturbances.

In this chapter, we tried to share with the readers our eight years' experience in researching the connection between vitamin B_6 and its influence on different kinds of psychotropic drug-induced movement disorders and mental state. Our serial research of this subject, including preliminary results and ongoing studies, suggest that vitamin B_6 has the ability to relieve symptoms of acute and tardive (delayed) psychotropic-induced movement disorders. The influence on psychotic symptoms in chronically resistant schizophrenic and schizoaffective patients was not confirmed, and further studies with enrolling subjects suffering from acute state and treatment with higher doses of the vitamin should be continued. Our long-time experience with using high doses of vitamin B_6 has brought us to the conclusion that a dose of 1,200 mg/day is safe. Throughout all of these years, we have not seen any neurotoxic side effects.

REFERENCES

[1] Barness LA, Tomarelli RM. Paul Gyorgy (1893-1976). A biographical sketch. *J. Nutr.* 1979; 109: 19-23.

[2] Henderson L, Hulse J. Vitamin B6: Relationship to tryptophan metabolism. Human Vitamin B6 Requirements: proceedings of a workshop. Washington, DC: National Academy of Sciences, 1978; 21-36.

[3] Roman GC. Nutritional disorders of the nervous system. In: Shils ME, ed. *Modern Nutrition in Health and Disease*, 10th ed. Baltimore: Lippincott Williams and Wilkins, 2006; 1363-1380.

[4] Edgar CE, El Sadr MM, Macrae TF. The water-soluble B-vitamins. The preparation from liver of fractions containing the same dietary essential factors for the rat as yeast eluate fraction and yeast filtrate fraction. *Biochem. J.* 1938; 32: 2225-2230.

[5] Sauberlich HE. Vitamin B-6 (pyridoxine). In: Sauberlich HE, ed. *Laboratory Tests for the Assessment of Nutritional Status*, 2nd ed, vol 71–102. Boca Raton: CRC Press, 1999.

[6] Clayton PT. B(6)-responsive disorders: A model of vitamin dependency. *J. Inherit. Metab. Dis.* 2006; 29: 317-26.

[7] Bauernfeid JC, Miller ON. Vitamin B6: nutritional and pharmaceutical usage, stability, bioavailability, antagonists, and safety. Human Vitamin B6 Requirements: proceedings of a workshop. Washington, DC: National Academy of Sciences, 1978; 78-110.

[8] McCormick DB. Vitamin B6. In: Young VR, ed. *Modern Nutrition in Health and Disease*. Philadelphia: Lea and Febiger, 1988; 376-382.

[9] Holman P. Pyridoxine - vitamin B-6. *J. Austral. Coll. Nutr. Environment Med.* 1995; 14: 5-16.

[10] Borenstein B, Lachance PA. Effects of processing and preparation on the nutritive value of foods. In: Young VR, ed. *Modern Nutrition in Health and Disease*, 7th ed. Philadelphia: Lea and Febiger, 1988; 673-684.

[11] U.S. Department of Agriculture, Agricultural Research Service. 1999. USDA Nutrient Database for Standard Reference, Release 13. Nutrient Data Laboratory Home Page, http://www.nal.usda.gov/fnic/foodcomp

[12] Leklem JE. Vitamin B6. In: Machlin LJ, ed. *Handbooks of Vitamins*. New York: Marcel Dekker, 1991; 341-392.

[13] Leklem JE. Vitamin B6. In: Shils ME, Olson JA, Shike M, et al., eds. *Modern Nutrition in Health and Disease*, 9th ed. Baltimore: Williams andWilkins, 1999; 413-421.

[14] Leklem JE. Vitamin B-6: a status report. *J. Nutr.* 1990; 120 Suppl 11: 1503-7.

[15] Institute of Medicine, Food and Nutrition Board. *Vitamin B6. Dietary Reference Intakes for Thiamine, Riboflavin, Niacin, Vitamin B6, Folate, Vitamin B12, Pantothenic Acid, Biotin, and Choline*. Washington, DC: National Academy Press, 1998; 150-195.

[16] Lerner V, Miodownik C, Kaptsan A, Cohen H, Matar M, Loewenthal U, Kotler M. Vitamin B6 in the treatment of tardive dyskinesia: a double-blind, placebo-controlled, crossover study. *Am. J. Psychiatry* 2001; 158: 1511-4.

[17] Miodownik C, Lerner V, Cohen H, Kotler M. Serum vitamin B6 in schizophrenic and schizoaffective patients with and without tardive dyskinesia. *Clin. Neuropharmacol.* 2000; 23: 212-5.

[18] Sener U, Zorlu Y, Karaguzel O, Ozdamar O, Coker I, Topbas M. Effects of common anti-epileptic drug monotherapy on serum levels of homocysteine, vitamin B12, folic acid and vitamin B6. *Seizure* 2006; 15: 79-85.

[19] Ubbink JB, Delport R, Becker PJ, Bissbort S. Evidence of a theophylline-induced vitamin B6 deficiency caused by noncompetitive inhibition of pyridoxal kinase. *J. Lab. Clin. Med.* 1989; 113: 15-22.

[20] Goodman LS, Gilman A. *The Pharmacologic Basis of Therapeutics*, 8 ed, Vol. II. New York: McGraw-Hill, 1992.

[21] Bender DA. Non-nutritional uses of vitamin B6. *Br. J. Nutr.* 1999; 81: 7-20.

[22] Lumeng L. The role of acetaldehyde in mediating the deleterious effect of ethanol on pyridoxal 5'-phosphate metabolism. *J. Clin. Invest* 1978; 62: 286-93.

[23] Schumann K. Interactions between drugs and vitamins at advanced age. *Int. J. Vitam. Nutr. Res.* 1999; 69: 173-8.

[24] Hansson O, Sillanpaa M. Letter: Pyridoxine and serum concentration of phenytoin and phenobarbitone. *Lancet* 1976; 1: 256.

[25] Pfeiffer CC. *Mental and Elemental Nutrients*. New Canaan, Connecticut: Keats Publishing, Inc, 1975.

[26] Marks J. *A Guide to the Vitamins: Their Role in Health and Disease.* London: MRP Medical and Technical Publishing Co. Ltd, 1979.

[27] Braestrup C, Nielsen M. Anxiety. *Lancet* 1982; 2: 1030-4.

[28] Mooney M. Vitamin and mineral doses: Safety and effectiveness. Access: 2002, www.supernutritionusa.com/vitamin.safety.doses9-02.pdf.

[29] Schaumburg H, Kaplan J, Windebank A, Vick N, Rasmus S, Pleasure D, Brown MJ. Sensory neuropathy from pyridoxine abuse. A new megavitamin syndrome. *N Engl. J. Med.* 1983; 309: 445-8.

[30] McLachlan RS, Brown WF. Pyridoxine dependent epilepsy with iatrogenic sensory neuronopathy. *Can. J. Neurol. Sci.* 1995; 22: 50-1.

[31] Berger AR, Schaumburg HH, Schroeder C, Apfel S, Reynolds R. Dose response, coasting, and differential fiber vulnerability in human toxic neuropathy: a prospective study of pyridoxine neurotoxicity. *Neurology* 1992; 42: 1367-70.

[32] Hausman P. The Right Dose: How to Take Vitamins and Minerals Safely. Emmaus, Pennsylvania: Rodale Press, 1987.

[33] Dalton K, Dalton M. Debate continues on vitamin B6 [letter] [see comments]. *Lancet* 1998; 352: 62.

[34] Marks J. Debate continues on vitamin B6 [letter]. *Lancet* 1998; 352: 63.

[35] Wang HS, Kuo MF, Chou ML, Hung PC, Lin KL, Hsieh MY, Chang MY. Pyridoxal phosphate is better than pyridoxine for controlling idiopathic intractable epilepsy. *Arch Dis. Child* 2005; 90: 512-5.

[36] Rimland B. Vitamin B6 (and magnesium) in the treatment of autism. *Autism Research Review International* 1987: 3.

[37] Miodownik C, Witztum E, Lerner V. Lithium-induced tremor treated with vitamin B6: a preliminary case series. *Int. J. Psychiatry in Medicine* 2002; 32: 103-108.

[38] Lerner V, Bergman J, Statsenko N, Miodownik C. Vitamin b(6) treatment in acute neuroleptic-induced akathisia: a randomized, double-blind, placebo-controlled study. *J. Clin. Psychiatry* 2004; 65: 1550-4.

[39] Miodownik C, Lerner V, Statsenko N, Dwolatzky T, Nemets B, Berzak E, Bergman J. Vitamin B6 versus mianserin and placebo in acute neuroleptic-induced akathisia: a randomized, double-blind, controlled study. *Clin. Neuropharmacol.* 2006; 29: 68-72.

[40] Lerner V, Miodownik C, Kaptsan A, Bersudsky Y, Libov I, Sela B-A, Witztum E. Vitamin B6 treatment for tardive dyskinesia: A randomized double-blind, placebo-controlled, crossover study. (submitted).

[41] Rudman D, Williams PJ. Megadose vitamins. Use and misuse. *N Engl. J. Med.* 1983; 309: 488-90.

[42] Snell EE. Summary of session I and some notes on the metabolism of vitamin B6. *Vitam. Horm.* 1964; 22: 485-94.

[43] Rimland B, Callaway E, Dreyfus P. The effect of high doses of vitamin B6 on autistic children: a double-blind crossover study. *Am. J. Psychiatry* 1978; 135: 472-5.

[44] Lelord G, Muh JP, Barthelemy C, Martineau J, Garreau B, Callaway E. Effects of pyridoxine and magnesium on autistic symptoms--initial observations. *J. Autism Dev. Disord.* 1981; 11: 219-30.

[45] Martineau J, Barthelemy C, Lelord G. Long-term effects of combined vitamin B6-magnesium administration in an autistic child. *Biological Psychiatry* 1986; 21: 511-8.

[46] Martineau J, Barthelemy C, Garreau B, Lelord G. Vitamin B6, magnesium, and combined B6-Mg: therapeutic effects in childhood autism. *Biological Psychiatry* 1985; 20: 467-78.

[47] Agbayewa MO, Bruce VM, Siemens V. Pyridoxine, ascorbic acid and thiamine in Alzheimer and comparison subjects. *Can. J. Psychiatry*. Revue Canadienne De Psychiatrie 1992; 37: 661-2.

[48] Colgan M, Colgan L. Do nutrient supplements and dietary changes affect learning and emotional reactions of children with learning difficulties? A controlled series of 16 cases. *Nutrition and Health* 1984; 3: 69-77.

[49] Frye PE, Arnold LE. Persistent amphetamine-induced compulsive rituals: response to pyridoxine(B6). *Biol. Psychiatry* 1981; 16: 583-7.

[50] Emmanuel NP, Lydiard RB, Reynolds RD, Roberts J, Johnson M, Mintzer O, Ballenger JC. Plasma pyridoxal phosphate in anxiety disorders. *Biol. Psychiatry* 1994; 36: 606-8.

[51] Wyatt KM, Dimmock PW, Jones PW, Shaughn O'Brien PM. Efficacy of vitamin B-6 in the treatment of premenstrual syndrome: systematic review. *BMJ* 1999; 318: 1375-81.

[52] Bucci L. Pyridoxine and schizophrenia. *Br. J. Psychiatry* 1973; 122: 240.

[53] Brooks SC, D'Angelo L, Chalmeta A, Ahern G, Judson JH. An unusual schizophrenic illness responsive to pyridoxine HCl (B6) subsequent to phenothiazine and butyrophenone toxicities. *Biological Psychiatry* 1983; 18: 1321-8.

[54] DeVeaugh-Geiss J, Manion L. High-dose pyridoxine in tardive dyskinesia. *J. Clin. Psychiatry* 1978; 39: 573-575.

[55] Tkacz C. A preventive measure for tardive dyskinesia [letter]. *J. Int. Acad. Preventive Med.* 1984; 8: 5.

[56] Devaux A. Dyskinesies tardives: role de la pyridoxine dans la prevention. *Semin. Hop. Paris* 1987; 63: 1476-1480.

[57] Sandyk R, Pardeshi, R. Pyridoxine improves drug-induced parkinsonism and psychosis in a schizophrenic patient. *Int. J. Neurosci.* 1990; 52(3-4): 225-232.

[58] Freeman JM, Finkelstein JD, Mudd SH. Folate-responsive homocystinuria and "schizophrenia". A defect in methylation due to deficient 5,10-methylenetetrahydrofolate reductase activity. *N. Engl. J. Med.* 1975; 292: 491-6.
[59] Petrie WM, Ban TA, Ananth JV. The use of nicotinic acid and pyridoxine in the treatment of schizophrenia. *Int. Pharmacopsychiatry* 1981; 16: 245-50.
[60] Lerner V, Liberman M. Movement disorders and psychotic symptoms treated with pyridoxine: a case report [letter]. *J. Clin. Psychiatry* 1998; 59: 623-4.
[61] Adams JB, George F, Audhya T. Abnormally high plasma levels of vitamin B6 in children with autism not taking supplements compared to controls not taking supplements. *J. Altern. Complement Med.* 2006; 12: 59-63.
[62] Botticher B, Botticher D. A new HPLC-method for the simultaneous determination of B1-, B2- and B6-vitamers in serum and whole blood. *Int. J. Vitam. Nutr. Res.* 1987; 57: 273-8.
[63] Rybak ME, Jain RB, Pfeiffer CM. Clinical vitamin B6 analysis: an interlaboratory comparison of pyridoxal 5'-phosphate measurements in serum. *Clin. Chem.* 2005; 51: 1223-31.
[64] Martineau J, Garreau B, Barthelemy C, Callaway E, Lelord G. Effects of vitamin B6 on averaged evoked potentials in infantile autism. *Biol. Psychiatry* 1981; 16: 627-41.
[65] Pfeiffer CC. The schizophrenias '76. *Biol. Psychiatry* 1976; 11: 773-5.
[66] Cruz R, Vogel WH. Pyroluria: a poor marker in chronic schizophrenia. *Am. J. Psychiatry* 1978; 135: 1239-40.
[67] Agnati LF, Genedani S, Rasio G, Galantucci M, Saltini S, Filaferro M, Franco R, Mora F, Ferre S, Fuxe K. Studies on homocysteine plasma levels in Alzheimer's patients. Relevance for neurodegeneration. *J. Neural Transm.* 2005; 112: 163-9.
[68] Muntjewerff JW, van der Put N, Eskes T, Ellenbroek B, Steegers E, Blom H, Zitman F. Homocysteine metabolism and B-vitamins in schizophrenic patients: low plasma folate as a possible independent risk factor for schizophrenia. *Psychiatry Res.* 2003; 121: 1-9.
[69] Levine J, Stahl Z, Sela BA, Ruderman V, Shumaico O, Babushkin I, Osher Y, Bersudsky Y, Belmaker RH. Homocysteine-reducing strategies improve symptoms in chronic schizophrenic patients with hyperhomocysteinemia. *Biol. Psychiatry* 2006; 60: 265-9.
[70] Ananth JV, Ban TA, Lehmann HE. Potentiation of therapeutic effects of nicotinic acid by pyridoxine in chronic schizophrenics. *Can. Psychiatr. Assoc. J.* 1973; 18: 377-83.
[71] Ban TA, Lehmann HE, Deutsch M. Negative findings with megavitamins in schizophrenic patients: preliminary report. *Communications in Psychopharmacology* 1977; 1: 119-22.
[72] Lerner V, Miodownik C, Kaptsan A, Cohen H, Loewenthal U, Kotler M. Vitamin B6 as add-on treatment in chronic schizophrenic and schizoaffective patients: a double-blind, placebo-controlled study. *J. Clin. Psychiatry* 2002; 63: 54-8.
[73] Lerner V, Miodownik C, Kaptsan A, Cohen H, Matar M, Loewenthal U, Kotler M. Vitamin B6 in the treatment of tardive dyskinesia: a double-blind, placebo-controlled, crossover study. *Am. J. Psychiatry* 2001; 158: 1511-1514.
[74] Wei IL, Huang YH, Wang GS. Vitamin B6 deficiency decreases the glucose utilization in cognitive brain structures of rats. *J. Nutr. Biochem.* 1999; 10: 525-31.
[75] Guilarte TR. Vitamin B6 and cognitive development: recent research findings from human and animal studies. *Nutr. Rev.* 1993; 51: 193-8.

[76] Mulder C, Scheltens P, Barkhof F, Gundy C, Verstraeten RA, de Leeuw FE. Low vitamin B6 levels are associated with white matter lesions in Alzheimer's disease. *J. Am. Geriatr. Soc.* 2005; 53: 1073-4.

[77] Malouf R, Grimley Evans J. The effect of vitamin B6 on cognition. *Cochrane Database Syst. Rev.* 2003: CD004393.

[78] Selhub J, Bagley LC, Miller J, Rosenberg IH. B vitamins, homocysteine, and neurocognitive function in the elderly. *Am. J. Clin. Nutr.* 2000; 71: 614S-620S.

[79] Riggs KM, Spiro A, 3rd, Tucker K, Rush D. Relations of vitamin B-12, vitamin B-6, folate, and homocysteine to cognitive performance in the Normative Aging Study. *Am. J. Clin. Nutr.* 1996; 63: 306-14.

[80] Sandyk R. L-tryptophan in neuropsychiatric disorders: a review. *Int. J. Neurosci.* 1992; 67: 127-44.

[81] Dupuis B, Catteau J, Dumon JP, Libert C, Petit H. Comparison of propranolol, sotalol, and betaxolol in the treatment of neuroleptic-induced akathisia. *Am. J. Psychiatry* 1987; 144: 802-5.

[82] American Psychiatric Association. *Diagnostic and Statistical Manual of Mental Disorders*, 4th ed. Washington, DC: American Psychiatric Association, 1994.

[83] Sachdev P. The epidemiology of drug-induced akathisia: Part I. Acute akathisia. *Schizophr. Bull.* 1995; 21: 431-49.

[84] Halliday J, Farrington S, Macdonald S, MacEwan T, Sharkey V, McCreadie R. Nithsdale Schizophrenia Surveys 23: movement disorders. 20-year review. *Br. J. Psychiatry* 2002; 181: 422-7.

[85] Adler LA, Angrist B, Reiter S, Rotrosen J. Neuroleptic-induced akathisia: a review. *Psychopharmacology* (Berl) 1989; 97: 1-11.

[86] Poyurovsky M, Weizman A. Serotonin-based pharmacotherapy for acute neuroleptic-induced akathisia: a new approach to an old problem. *Br. J. Psychiatry* 2001; 179: 4-8.

[87] Barnes TR. A rating scale for drug-induced akathisia. *Br. J. Psychiatry* 1989; 154: 672-6.

[88] Hansen L. A critical review of akathisia, and its possible association with suicidal behaviour. *Hum. Psychopharmacol.* 2001; 16: 495-505.

[89] Kim JH, Byun HJ. Prevalence and characteristics of subjective akathisia, objective akathisia, and mixed akathisia in chronic schizophrenic subjects. *Clin. Neuropharmacol.* 2003; 26: 312-6.

[90] Kapur S, Remington G. Serotonin-dopamine interaction and its relevance to schizophrenia. *Am. J. Psychiatry* 1996; 153: 466-76.

[91] Poyurovsky M, Fuchs C, Weizman A. Low-dose mianserin in treatment of acute neuroleptic-induced akathisia. *J. Clin. Psychopharmacol.* 1998; 18: 253-4.

[92] Poyurovsky M, Weizman A. Serotonin antagonists and neuroleptic-induced extrapyramidal symptoms. *Isr. J. Psychiatry Relat. Sci.* 1998; 35: 70-1.

[93] Poyurovsky M, Shardorodsky M, Fuchs C, Schneidman M, Weizman A. Treatment of neuroleptic-induced akathisia with the 5-HT2 antagonist mianserin. Double-blind, placebo-controlled study. *Br. J. Psychiatry* 1999; 174: 238-42.

[94] Fischel T, Hermesh H, Aizenberg D, Zemishlany Z, Munitz H, Benjamini Y, Weizman A. Cyproheptadine versus propranolol for the treatment of acute neuroleptic-induced akathisia: a comparative double-blind study. *J. Clin. Psychopharmacol.* 2001; 21: 612-5.

[95] Miller CH, Fleischhacker WW, Ehrmann H, Kane JM. Treatment of neuroleptic induced akathisia with the 5-HT2 antagonist ritanserin. *Psychopharmacol. Bull.* 1990; 26: 373-6.

[96] Weiss D, Aizenberg D, Hermesh H, Zemishlany Z, Munitz H, Radwan M, Weizman A. Cyproheptadine treatment in neuroleptic-induced akathisia. *Br. J. Psychiatry* 1995; 167: 483-6.

[97] Burton K. The treatment of tremor. *Med. J. Australia* 1987; 147: 503-506.

[98] Kane J, Rifkin A, Quitkin F, Klein DF. Extrapyramidal side effects with lithium treatment. *Am. J. Psychiatry* 1978; 135: 851-3.

[99] Tyrer P, Alexander MS, Regan A, Lee I. An extrapyramidal syndrome after lithium therapy. *Br. J. Psychiatry* 1980; 136: 191-4.

[100] Tyrer P, Lee I, Trotter C. Physiological characteristics of tremor after chronic lithium therapy. *Br. J. Psychiatry* 1981; 139: 59-61.

[101] Burke RE. Tardive dyskinesia: current clinical issues. *Neurology* 1984; 34: 1348-53.

[102] Cummings JL, Wirshing WC. Recognition and differential diagnosis of tardive dyskinesia. *Int. J. Psychiatry Med.* 1989; 19: 133-44.

[103] Klawans H. Recognition and diagnosis of tardive dyskinesia. *J. Clin. Psychiatry* 1985; 46: 3-7.

[104] Fernandez HH, Friedman JH. Classification and treatment of tardive syndromes. *Neurologist* 2003; 9: 16-27.

[105] Sachdev PS. The current status of tardive dyskinesia. *Aust. N. Z. J. Psychiatry* 2000; 34: 355-69.

[106] Tarsy D. History and definition of tardive dyskinesia. *Clinical Neuropharmacology* 1983; 6: 91-9.

[107] Stacy M, Jankovic J. Tardive tremor. *Mov. Disord* 1992; 7: 53-7.

[108] Chouinard G. New nomenclature for drug-induced movement disorders including tardive dyskinesia. *J. Clin. Psychiatry* 2004; 65 Suppl 9: 9-15.

[109] Storey E, Lloyd J. Tardive tremor. *Mov. Dis.* 1997; 12: 808-10.

[110] Kane JM. Tardive Dyskinesia. In: Jeste DV, Wyatt RJ, eds. Neuropsychiatric Movement Disorders. Washington, DC: American Psychiatric Press, 1984; 68-95.

[111] Jeste DV, Caliguiri MP. Tardive dyskinesia. *Schizophr. Bull.* 1993; 19: 303-315.

[112] Kane JM, Woerner M, Lieberman J. Tardive dyskinesia. Prevalence, incidence and risk factor. *J. Clin. Psychopharmacology* 1988; 8: 52-56.

[113] Barnes TR, McPhillips MA. Novel antipsychotics, extrapyramidal side effects and tardive dyskinesia. *Int. Clin. Psychopharmacol.* 1998; 13 Suppl 3: S49-57.

[114] Caroff SN, Mann SC, Campbell EC, Sullivan KA. Movement disorders associated with atypical antipsychotic drugs. *J. Clin. Psychiatry* 2002; 63 Suppl 4: 12-9.

[115] Glazer WM. Expected incidence of tardive dyskinesia associated with atypical antipsychotics. *J. Clin. Psychiatry* 2000; 61 Suppl 4: 21-6.

[116] Silberbauer C. Risperidone-induced tardive dyskinesia. *Pharmacopsychiatry* 1998; 31: 68-9.

[117] Ananth J, Kenan J. Tardive dyskinesia associated with olanzapine monotherapy. J. *Clin. Psychiatry* 1999; 60: 870.

[118] Ghelber D, Belmaker RH. Tardive dyskinesia with quetiapine. *Am. J. Psychiatry* 1999; 156: 796-7.

[119] Herran A, Vazquez-Barquero JL. Tardive dyskinesia associated with olanzapine. *Ann. Intern. Med.* 1999; 131: 72.
[120] Molho ES, Factor SA. Possible tardive dystonia resulting from clozapine therapy. *Mov. Disord.* 1999; 14: 873-4.
[121] Bassitt DP, de Souza Lobo Garcia L. Risperidone-induced tardive dyskinesia. *Pharmacopsychiatry* 2000; 33: 155-6.
[122] Bella VL, Piccoli F. Olanzapine-induced tardive dyskinesia. *Br. J. Psychiatry* 2003; 182: 81-2.
[123] Ananth J, Burgoyne KS, Niz D, Smith M. Tardive dyskinesia in 2 patients treated with ziprasidone. *J. Psychiatry Neurosci.* 2004; 29: 467-9.
[124] Keck ME, Muller MB, Binder EB, Sonntag A, Holsboer F. Ziprasidone-related tardive dyskinesia. *Am. J. Psychiatry* 2004; 161: 175-6.
[125] Ertugrul A, Demir B. Clozapine-induced tardive dyskinesia: a case report. *Prog. Neuropsychopharmacol. Biol. Psychiatry* 2005; 29: 633-5.
[126] Soares KV, McGrath JJ. The treatment of tardive dyskinesia--a systematic review and meta-analysis. *Schizophr. Res.* 1999; 39: 1-16.
[127] Dakshinamurti K, Paulose CS, Viswanathan M, Siow YL, Sharma SK, Bolster B. Neurobiology of pyridoxine. *Ann. N. Y. Acad. Sci.* 1990; 585: 128-44.
[128] Schaeffer MC, Cochary EF, Sadowski JA. Subtle abnormalities of gait detected early in vitamin B6 deficiency in aged and weanling rats with hind leg gait analysis. *J. Am. Coll. Nutr.* 1990; 9: 120-7.
[129] Paulson GW. Use of pyridoxine in chorea. [letter]. *Am. J. Psychiatry* 1971; 127: 1091.
[130] Lerner V, Kaptsan A, Miodownik C, Kotler M. Vitamin B6 in treatment of tardive dyskinesia: a preliminary case series study. *Clin. Neuropharmacol.* 1999; 22: 241-3.
[131] American Psychiatric Association. Diagnostic and Statistical Manual of Mental Disorders, 4, Text Revision ed. Washington, DC: American Psychiatric Association, 2000.
[132] Chouinard G, Ross-Chouinard A, Annable L, Jones B. Extrapyramidal Symptom Rating Scale. *Can. J. Neurol. Sci.* (abstract) 1980; 7: 233.
[133] Chouinard G, Margolese HC. Manual for the Extrapyramidal Symptom Rating Scale (ESRS). *Schizophr. Res.* 2005; 76: 247-65.

In: New Hope for Mental Disturbances
Editors: Vladimir Lerner and Chanoch Meodownik

ISBN 978-1-60692-691-8

Chapter 3

VITAMIN B_6 IN TREATING MOOD AND RELATED DISORDERS

Chanoch Miodownik [1] and Vladimir Lerner
Division of Psychiatry, Ministry of Health Be'er Sheva Mental Health Center,
Faculty of Health Sciences Ben-Gurion University of the Negev, Be'er-Sheva, Israel

ABSTRACT

Depression is one of the frequent and disabling conditions in the world. About 10% of the population suffers from a kind of clinical depression. Sometimes it is difficult to differ whether it is a primary problem, but during the last decades more have been known about the combinations of depressive states and deficiency of at least one nutrient. Mood disorders are associated with heterogeneous dysregulation of the biogenic amines. Norepinephrine and serotonin have an important role in etiology of depression. The cholinergic, dopaminergic, and GABA system have also been associated with depression.

One of the possible explanations for the aetiology of depression, related to serotonin theory, is that vitamin B6 which is a key enzyme involved in the synthesis of different neurotransmitters and its deficiency may lead to appearance of depression.

Depression is not a crime. But it plummets a person into an abyss deeper than any crime could reach. Rabbi Menachem M. Schneerson [1]

INTRODUCTION

Depression strikes about 17 million American adults each year – more than cancer, AIDS, or coronary heart disease – according to the National Institute of Mental Health

1 Corresponding author: Chanoch Miodownik, Faculty of Health Sciences, Ben Gurion University of the Negev and Psychiatric Department at Be'er Sheva Mental Health Center. Mail address: Be'er Sheva Mental Health Center, PO Box 4600, Be'er Sheva 84170, Israel, Tel.: +972 8 6401404; Fax: +972 8 6401491; Email: chanoch_m@yahoo.com.

(NIMH). An estimated 15 percent of chronic depression cases end in suicide. Women are twice as likely as men to be affected. At any given time, 8% to 10% of the population suffers from some form of clinical depression; almost 70% of these individuals are women. It looks like depression is already the world's fourth largest cause of disability, and is expected to be second in about 10 years [2].

Left untreated, depression can result in years of needless pain for both the depressed person and his or her family. According to the National Depressive and Manic Depressive Association, total cost of depression in the United States is estimated approximately about $43 billion a year, due in large part to absenteeism from work, lost productivity, and medical costs.

According to the American Psychiatric Association (APA), 80 to 90 percent of all cases can be treated effectively. However, two-thirds of the people suffering from depression don't get the help they need.

Traditionally, the role of B vitamins in mental health was limited to recognition of the manifestations of psychiatric symptoms in thiamine, folate, B_{12}, and B_6 deficiencies, and appropriate replacement. A number of studies have examined the correlation between folate levels and psychiatric disorders, [7] prominent among these is the treatment of depression [8]. From the B vitamin replenishment literature grew scientific inquiry into the role of vitamin B_6 as treatment, both adjuvant and primary, for depression. Reported here is the result of a review examining the therapeutic efficacy of vitamin B_6 for depression and related disorders

Many famous names of artists, composers, writers, politicians each of them was a virtuoso in his area. Ludwig von Beethoven (1770-1827), Edgar Allen Poe *(1809-1849),* Robert Schumann *(1810-1856),* Mark Twain (1835-1910), Vincent van Gogh *(1853-1890),* Abraham Lincoln (1861-1865), Theodore Roosevelt (1901-1909), Sir Winston Churchill *(1874-1965),* Georgia O'Keefe (1887-1986), and many others. Each of them was from different dimension, but in fact, these historical figures also had a much more personal common experience. In addition to their virtuosity had to battle with the debilitating illness of depression which affected their life in sometimes changed the whole history of their life and sometimes of the nations [3-6].

It is common for people to speak of how "depressed" they are. However, the occasional sadness everyone feels due to life's situations like disappointments, separations, bereavement etc, is very different from the serious illness caused by a brain disorder. All these conditions produce reactive depression which can be temporary and self limited. Such adjustment reactions may be healed without any professional psychiatric intervention, and conversation psychotherapy may be enough. On the opposite side, depressive disorders profoundly impair the ability to function in everyday life by affecting moods, thoughts, occupational, social behaviors, and physical well-being and even a threatening of life. This disturbance may long for months or even years in untreated cases. That the reason for recommendation to treat every moderate to severe depressive patient in order to shorten the course of the illness.

It is not a surprise that one of the most common features in people who suffer from depression and other mental disorders is their poor dietary habits. It is difficult to differ what is the primary problem, but there are documented observations about the combinations of depressive states and deficiency of at least one nutrient. A deficiency of any single nutrient can alter brain function and lead to mood changes, anxiety, and other mental disorders. In treating depression, it is important to follow up and control of food intake which influence the brain chemical input.

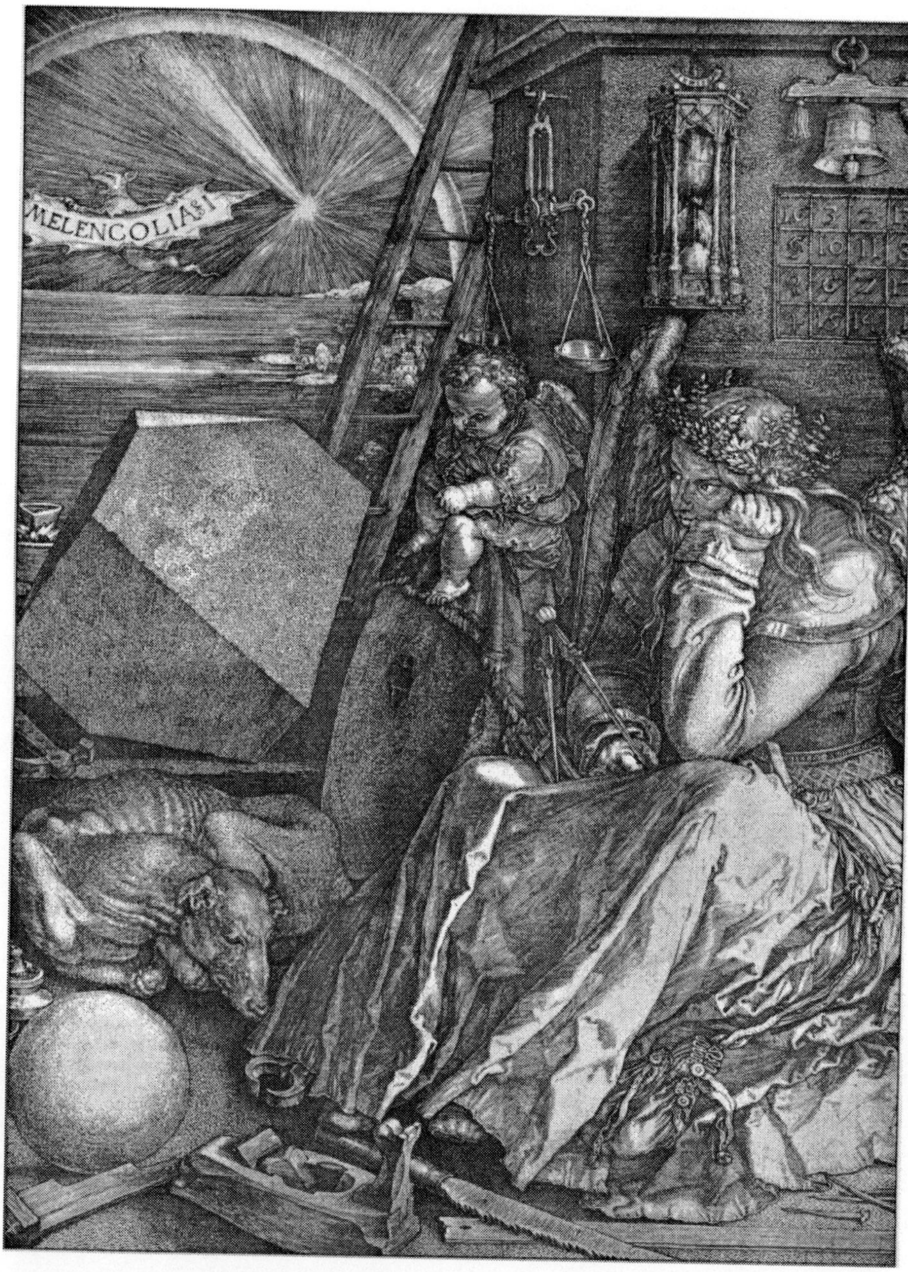

Figure 1. Albrecht Dürer "Melancholy" (1514).

The depressive phenomenon is well known for ages. King Saul suffered from depression and needed a spiritual medicine given by David who played for him a lyre music. The famous artist Albrecht Dürer in 1514 painted a picture called “Melancholia” in which he presented a portrait of his own temperament as artist. According to his imagination melancholy has wings and from her belt hang keys and a money bag, symbolizing power and wealth. She is surrounded by measuring instruments. A panel of 'magic' numbers is above her head (they add up to 34 in all directions). At her feet are the tools that can fashion the material world. Yet she does nothing: lost in thought, she turns away from the light (Figure 1).

VITAMIN B_6 AND DEPRESSION

Clinical Vignette

Mr. A 37-year-old, a Hi-Tech engineer, married and father to 3 kids. He came to the mental health clinic and complained on decreased mood, anxiety, fatigue and loss of energy, general somatic discomfort, sleep disturbances and decreased occupational ability even though he continued working. Although he was an excessive book reader, during last month prior his request for help, he felt that his concentration became difficult and even TV movies were difficult for him to be seen. His appetite was bad; he could not enjoy his usual preferred goodies, and lost about 5 kg in weight during 2 months. He continued having a sexual activity, but his interest was diminished with less pleasure. The patient had no history of drug or alcohol abuse.

Mental status: Mr. A was well appeared and cooperative. His affect was quite sad. His speech was coherent and there were no thought disturbances or any other signs of psychosis. He totally denied suicidal ideas, in the contrary he asked for help in order to improve his quality of life.

The whole anamnesis led to the diagnosis of depression. SSRI drug was prescribed for him. He took it for about two months, without any subjective feeling of improvement, instead he complained on vomiting and abdominal pain. Exchanging this treatment to SNRI preparation did not have better influence. Since the patient was almost desperate he stopped the medication and sought help in a naturopathic clinic. The naturopath suggested him to start taking 500 mg/day of vitamin B_6*. A month later his mood was improved and gradually became euthymic. After six months, while he returned to his baseline occupation and social activities, he stopped the vitamin* B_6 *treatment. Unfortunately, just three months later, all the depressive symptoms came back. In this point of time, Mr. A came to our clinic. This time he was not excited to hear about conventional antidepressant treatment, therefore vitamin* B_6 *was prescribed for him in the same dose as before. In about a month his condition was better and he continued with this vitamin therapy.*

The experience with this patient attracted our attention to the possibility that vitamin B_6 apparently has an antidepressive property. That is the reason why we began to collect data regarding relationship between vitamin B_6 and its influence on depressive state and related conditions.

Vitamin B_6, or pyridoxine as its active derivate pyridoxal 5'-phosphate (PLP), is a cofactor for enzymes that convert L-tryptophan to serotonin and L-tyrosine to norepinephrine. It is essential in the manufacture of all monoamines from amino acids.

Bender and Totoe [9] found that high doses of vitamin B_6 (10 mg/kg body weight) led to decreased oxidative metabolism of tryptophan in rats. They also found increased plasma concentration of tryptophan, and increased uptake of tryptophan into the brain, leading to an increased rate of serotonin turnover. The authors' conclusion was that vitamin B_6 supplements might be a useful adjunct to tryptophan for the treatment of depression. It is likely that the impairment of tryptophan oxidation was the result of reduced induction of tryptophan dioxygenase by glucocorticoid hormones in the presence of high concentrations of PLP.

Mood disorders are associated with heterogeneous dysregulation of the biogenic amines. Norepinephrine and serotonin have an important role in etiology of depression. The cholinergic, dopaminergic, and GABA system have also been associated with depression.

One of the possible explanations for the aetiology of depression, related to serotonin theory, is that vitamin B_6 deficiency may cause a reduction in formation of the neurotransmitters - serotonin and catecholamines. PLP-dependent aromatic amino acid decarboxylase is a key enzyme involved in the synthesis of these neurotransmitters. According to this fact, it has been suggested that supplementation of vitamin B_6 may increase aromatic amino acid decarboxylase activity, followed by raising of amine synthesis, which in its turn leads to antidepressive effect [10].

The serotonin deficiency hypothesis proposes a functional deficiency of serotonin in the brain as the main cause of depression. Khan [11] supports the existence of disturbances in the transportation of L-tryptophan through the blood–brain barrier and its conversion to serotonin, as well as decreased density in serotonin uptake sites. Dakshinamurti and colleagues [12] reported a low brain concentration of serotonin, but not catecholamines, in vitamin B_6-deficient rats. Siow and Dakshinarnurti [13] found reduced decarboxylase activity towards 5-hydroxy-tryptophan, but not dopa (3-hydroxytyrosine), in the brains of vitamin B_6-deficient animals. The decarboxylase undergoes mechanism-dependent inactivation in the presence of serotonin, and may thus be more susceptible to inactivation in serotoninergic neurons than in catecholaminergic neurons. It is unlikely that it explains the differential effect of vitamin B_6 deficiency on serotonin and catecholamine formation, since the inactivation is the result of a covalent modification of the catalytic site, not the coenzyme, and is not reversed by incubation with PLP [14].

The noradrenergic hypothesis posits various abnormalities in the synthesis, release, and metabolism of norepinephrine as playing causal roles in depression [15]. Empirical support for this hypothesis has been found equivocal [11].

Since the active metabolite of vitamin B_6 (PLP), is a coenzyme in the tryptophan-serotonin pathway, a lack of vitamin B_6 might theoretically cause depression [16]. This theory is supported by studies demonstrating that depressed patients had low levels of vitamin B_6 [17-21]. Although low vitamin B_6 levels could be a result of dietary changes associated with depression, its deficiency could also be a contributing factor to the depression.

While severe vitamin B_6 deficiency is rare, marginal vitamin B_6 status may be relatively common. A study using a sensitive enzymatic assay suggested the presence of subtle vitamin B_6 deficiency among a group of 21 healthy individuals [22]. Few studies note the beneficial effect of add-on treatment with vitamin B_6 on depression as a part of premenstrual syndrome (PMS) - a condition of nervousness, irritability, emotional disturbance, headache and/or depression suffered by many women for up to 10 days before menstruation. Although the researches remain inconsistent [23, 24], it has to be mentioned that in all the reports and studies dealing with the efficacy of vitamin B_6 in PMS the doses of the medication were from 50 mg/day to maximum 500 mg/day. Kleijnen with coworkers [24] reviewed twelve placebo-controlled double-blind trials of vitamin B_6 in the PMS and concluded that the evidence for beneficial effects was weak. In three of the studies cited there was a significant beneficial effect of vitamin B_6 supplements: Abraham and Hargrove [25] used a dose of 500 mg/day, Hallman and Oreland [24] 300 mg/day and Barr [26] 100 mg/day. A further five studies yielded ambiguous results. Doll and colleagues [27] reported a significant beneficial effect of 50 mg/day on depression, irritability and tiredness, but none of the other premenstrual symptoms. Kendall and Schnurr [28] reported that 150 mg/day led to some improvement in dizziness, vomiting and behavioral changes, but considerable physical and affective symptoms remained. Williams and coworkers [29] showed an improvement for 82 % of subjects receiving 100 mg vitamin B_6 per day, and 70 % of those receiving placebo. Smallwood and colleagues [30] reported a positive trend but no statistical significance using 200 mg/day, and Stokes and Mendels [31] reported disappointing and 'not clear' results using 50 mg/day. The remaining four studies they reviewed reported no beneficial effects of doses of between 100 and 500 mg/day. The supplementation of vitamin B_6 works with positive results, although there is no evidence that women who suffer from PMS have any lower vitamin B_6 status than others, and the same about another gender related phenomenon as postpartum depression [10, 32-36]. There is no even one report of higher dose which may convert ambiguity of the results into more significant data. Anyway it is known that there is no direct correlation between the serum vitamin B_6 level and its brain level. Moreover, there are some studies showing that vitamin B_6 supplements could be effective in overcoming some of the side-effects of oral contraceptives in high dose have led to the use of vitamin B_6 in treatment of PMS. Depression is also a relatively common side effect of oral contraceptives. A double-blind research shows that women who were depressed and who have become depleted of vitamin B_6 while taking oral contraceptives typically responded to vitamin B_6 supplementation [37]. Other studies also confirm the efficacy of vitamin B_6 in such cases [20, 38].

Ooylan et al [39] found that mothers with vitamin B_6 intake greater than the median value had a significantly higher median pyridoxal level in their breast milk than did the mothers with intake below the median value. Vitamin B_6 is important for normal behavioral functioning of infants. The mothers' vitamin B_6 intake affects vitamin B_6 levels of breast milk and the need for consuming recommended levels of vitamin B_6 should be emphasized to all pregnant and lactating mothers. In a double-blind, crossover trial, women with vitamin B_6 deficiency improved after adding pyridoxine [37]. Women who were not deficient in the vitamin did not respond to supplementation [40].

Shiloh et al. describe preliminary results of an open-label study in which schizophrenic patients with co-morbid minor depression received pyridoxine 150 mg/day in addition to their anti-psychotic treatment for 4 consecutive weeks. The authors conclusion was that a subgroup of schizophrenic patients with comorbid minor depression may benefit from pyridoxine addition to their on-going anti-psychotic treatment [41].

Williams and coworkers in their review about treatment effect of vitamin B_6 for depression in general was not apparent. However, examination of papers addressing depression in pre-menopausal women only, reveals a consistent message about the value of using vitamin B_6 supplementation. The authors came into conclusion that further study of vitamin B_6 as independent and adjuvant therapy for hormone related depression in women is indicated [42].

Vitamin B_6 and Anxiety Disorders

Depression commonly appears as co-morbidity with related anxiety disorders (in more than 50%) [43]. For this reason it was interesting to find whether there is correlation between depression anxiety and vitamin B_6 serum levels. Hoes in his review concluded that a combination of tryptophan and B_6 may be effective in anxiety states [44]. Unfortunately this author used an idiosyncratic terminology which means unusual professional terms to describe anxiety states and their relationship to stress. It makes it difficult to arrive at definitive conclusions. Some authors who support the lactate hypothesis of panic disorder point out that vitamin B_6 supplementation may diminish the conversion of pyruvate to lactate by facilitating transamination reactions which would feed substrate into the Krebs cycle [45].

Some researchers found a low plasma level of PLP in patients with anxiety disorders [46]. This correlation was also found in animal models for hypertension in rats with the serum vitamin B_6 low level [47-50]. These results are not surprising as the connection between mental stress and arterial hypertension is known for a long time. Moreover, there are clues in animal experiments in which vitamin B_6 has an analgesic effect [51-53].

The explanation for these relations between all those mental disturbances is passing through serotonin and GABA which are decreased in conditions of vitamin B_6 deficiency. The imbalance of GABA and serotonin may induce exacerbation of dysphoria and its physiological consequences, pain perception, anxiety and even psychological stress following bereavement [54]. Ellis noticed that use of vitamin B_6 in doses of 100–300 mg daily in his clinical practice tended to have a favorable impact on dysphoric states [55].

SUMMARY

In the chapter above, we tried to summarize all the scientific materials regarding the use of vitamin B_6 in treating depression, anxiety and related disturbances. Viewed as a whole, meaningful treatment effect of vitamin B_6 for depression in general was not apparent. However, examination of papers addressing depression in pre-menopausal women only, reveals a consistent message about the value of using vitamin B_6 supplementation. In cases of depression as single diagnosis, vitamin B_6 was effective as augmentation of antidepressive medications. These studies indicate that vitamin B_6 supplementation may be considered as a valuable factor for a subset of depressed patients. Even more importantly, randomized controlled trials are justified and needed in order to show whether treatment with vitamin B_6 may improve symptoms of depression among individuals with low levels of vitamin B_6. Because of its role in monoamine metabolism, this vitamin should be investigated as a possible adjunctive treatment for patients with depression connected to different etiologies including hormone related depression in women also is needed [42].

REFERENCES

[1] Schneerson RMM. Bringing Heaven Down to Earth: Meditations and Everyday Wisdom from the Teachings of the Rebbe, Menachem Schneerson. Adams Media Corporation, 1999.

[2] Stahl SM. Essential Psychopharmacology: Neuroscientic Basis and Practical Applications, 2 ed. Cambridge: Cambridge University Press, 2000.

[3] Storr A. Churchill's Black Dog, Kafka's Mice, and Other Phenomena of the Human Mind. New York: Ballantine Books, 1990.

[4] Spivak M. Posmertnaya Diagnostika Genial'nosti [Posthumous Diagnosis of Genius]. Moscow: Agraf, 2001.

[5] Toole JF. Dementia in world leaders and its effects upon international events: the examples of Franklin D. Roosevelt and T. Woodrow Wilson. *Eur. J. Neurol.* 1999; 6: 115-9.

[6] Freeman H. The human brain and political behaviour. *Br. J. Psychiatry* 1991; 159: 19-32.

[7] Godfrey PS, Toone BK, Carney MW, Flynn TG, Bottiglieri T, Laundy M, Chanarin I, Reynolds EH. Enhancement of recovery from psychiatric illness by methylfolate. *Lancet* 1990; 336: 392-5.

[8] Abou-Saleh MT, Coppen A. Serum and red blood cell folate in depression. *Acta Psychiatr. Scand.* 1989; 80: 78-82.

[9] Bender DA, Totoe L. High doses of vitamin B6 in the rat are associated with inhibition of hepatic tryptophan metabolism and increased uptake of tryptophan into the brain. *J. Neurochem.* 1984; 43: 733-6.

[10] Bender DA. Non-nutritional uses of vitamin B6. *Br. J. Nutr.* 1999; 81: 7-20.

[11] Khan AU. Neurochemistry of Schizophrenia and Depression. Clovis, CA: A.J. Publisher, 1998.

[12] Dakshinamurti K, LeBlancq WD, Herchl R, Havlicek V. Nonparallel changes in brain monoamines of pyridoxine-deficient growing rats. *Exp. Brain Res.* 1976; 26: 355-66.

[13] Siow YL, Dakshinamurti K. Effect of pyridoxine deficiency on aromatic L-amino acid decarboxylase in adult rat brain. *Exp. Brain Res.* 1985; 59: 575-81.

[14] Bertoldi M, Moore PS, Maras B, Dominici P, Voltattorni CB. Mechanism-based inactivation of dopa decarboxylase by serotonin. *J. Biol. Chem.* 1996; 271: 23954-9.

[15] Schilderkraut JJ. The catecholamine hypothesis of affective disorders: A review of supporting evidence. *Am. J. Psychiatry* 1965; 122: 509-522.

[16] Bernstein AL. Vitamin B-6 in clinical neurology. *Ann. N Y Acad. Sci.* 1990; 585: 250-260.

[17] Carney MW, Williams DG, Sheffield BF. Thiamine and pyridoxine lack newly-admitted psychiatric patients. *Br. J. Psychiatry* 1979; 135: 249-54.

[18] Carney MW, Ravindran A, Rinsler MG, Williams DG. Thiamine, riboflavin and pyridoxine deficiency in psychiatric in-patients. *Br. J. Psychiatry* 1982; 141: 271-2.

[19] Stewart JW, Harrison W, Quitkin F, Baker H. Low B6 levels in depressed outpatients. *Biol. Psychiatry* 1984; 19: 613-6.

[20] Hvas AM, Juul S, Bech P, Nexo E. Vitamin B6 level is associated with symptoms of depression. *Psychother. Psychosom.* 2004; 73: 340-3.

[21] Nobbs BT. Letter: Pyridoxal phosphate status in clinical depression. *Lancet* 1974; 1: 405-6.

[22] Azuma J, Kishi T, Williams RH, Folkers K. Apparent deficiency of vitamin B6 in typical individuals who commonly serve as normal controls. *Res. Commun. Chem. Pathol. Pharmacol.* 1976; 14: 343-66.

[23] Gunn AD. Vitamin B6 and the premenstrual syndrome (PMS). *Int. J. Vitam. Nutr. Res. Suppl.* 1985; 27: 213-24.

[24] Kleijnen J, Ter Riet G, Knipschild P. Vitamin B6 in the treatment of the premenstrual syndrome--a review. *Br. J. Obstet Gynaecol.* 1990; 97: 847-52.

[25] Abraham GE, Hargrove JT. Effect of vitamin B6 on premenstrual symptomatology in women with premenstrual tension syndromes, a double-blind cross-over study. *Infertility* 1980; 3: 155-165.
[26] Barr W. Pyridoxine supplements in the premenstrual syndrome. *Practitioner* 1984; 228: 425-7.
[27] Doll H, Brown S, Thurston A, Vessey M. Pyridoxine (vitamin B6) and the premenstrual syndrome: a randomized crossover trial. *J. R Coll Gen. Pract.* 1989; 39: 364-8.
[28] Kendall KE, Schnurr PP. The effects of vitamin B6 supplementation on premenstrual symptoms. *Obstet Gynecol.* 1987; 70: 145-9.
[29] Williams MJ, Harris RI, Dean BC. Controlled trial of pyridoxine in the premenstrual syndrome. *J. Int. Med. Res.* 1985; 13: 174-9.
[30] Smallwood J, Ah-Kye D, Taylor I. Vitamin B6 in the treatment of pre-menstrual mastalgia. *Br. J. Clin. Pract.* 1986; 40: 532-3.
[31] Stokes J, Mendels J. Pyridoxine and premenstrual tension. Lancet 1972; 1: 1177-8.
[32] Livingston JE, MacLeod PM, Applegarth DA. Vitamin B6 status in women with postpartum depression. *Am. J. Clin. Nutr.* 1978; 31: 886-91.
[33] Miyake Y, Sasaki S, Yokoyama T, Tanaka K, Ohya Y, Fukushima W, Saito K, Ohfuji S, Kiyohara C, Hirota Y. Risk of postpartum depression in relation to dietary fish and fat intake in Japan: the Osaka Maternal and Child Health Study. *Psychol. Med.* 2006: 1-9.
[34] Ritchie CD, Singkamani R. Plasma pyridoxal 5'-phosphate in women with the premenstrual syndrome. *Hum. Nutr. Clin. Nutr.* 1986; 40: 75-80.
[35] van den Berg H, Louwerse ES, Bruinse HW, Thissen JT, Schrijver J. Vitamin B6 status of women suffering from premenstrual syndrome. *Hum. Nutr. Clin. Nutr.* 1986; 40: 441-50.
[36] Mira M, Stewart PM, Abraham SF. Vitamin and trace element status in premenstrual syndrome. *Am. J. Clin. Nutr.* 1988; 47: 636-41.
[37] Adams PW, Rose DP, Folkard J, Wynn V, Seed M, Strong R. Effect of pyridoxine hydrochloride (vitamin B 6) upon depression associated with oral contraception. *Lancet* 1973; 1: 899-904.
[38] Wyatt KM, Dimmock PW, Jones PW, Shaughn O'Brien PM. Efficacy of vitamin B-6 in the treatment of premenstrual syndrome: systematic review. *BMJ* 1999; 318: 1375-81.
[39] Ooylan LM, Hart S, Porter KB, Driskell JA. Vitamin B-6 content of breast milk and neonatal behavioral functioning. *J. Am. Diet. Assoc.* 2002; 102: 1433-8.
[40] Brown D, Gaby AR, Reichert R. Natural Remedies for Depression. Access: Nutrition Science News, 1999 http://www.newhope.com/nutritionsciencenews/NSNbacks/feb_99/depression.cfm?path=ex,
[41] Shiloh R, Weizman A, Weizer N, Dorfman-Etrog P, Munitz H. [Antidepressive effect of pyridoxine (vitamin B6) in neuroleptic-treated schizophrenic patients with co-morbid minor depression--preliminary open-label trial]. *Harefuah* 2001; 140: 369-73, 456.
[42] Williams AL, Cotter A, Sabina A, Girard C, Goodman J, Katz DL. The role for vitamin B-6 as treatment for depression: a systematic review. *Fam. Pract.* 2005; 22: 532-7.
[43] American Psychiatric Association. Diagnostic and Statistical Manual of Mental Disorders (DSM-IV-TR), 4, Text Revision ed. Washington, DC: American Psychiatric Association, 2000.

[44] Hoes MJ. Monoamines in psychiatry: the role of serotonin in depression, anxiety and stress. *Acta Psychiatr. Belg.* 1982; 82: 287-309.
[45] Buist RA. Anxiety neurosis: The lactate connection. *Int. Clin. Nutr. Rev.* 1985; 5: 1-4.
[46] Emmanuel NP, Lydiard RB, Reynolds RD, Roberts J, Johnson M, Mintzer O, Ballenger JC. Plasma pyridoxal phosphate in anxiety disorders. *Biol. Psychiatry* 1994; 36: 606-8.
[47] Dakshinamurti K, Paulose CS, Viswanathan M. Vitamin B6 and hypertension. *Ann. N Y Acad. Sci.* 1990; 585: 241-9.
[48] Dakshinamurti K, Lal KJ. Vitamins and hypertension. *World Rev. Nutr. Diet* 1992; 69: 40-73.
[49] Lal KJ, Dakshinamurti K. Calcium channels in vitamin B6 deficiency-induced hypertension. *J. Hypertens.* 1993; 11: 1357-62.
[50] Lal KJ, Dakshinamurti K, Thliveris J. The effect of vitamin B6 on the systolic blood pressure of rats in various animal models of hypertension. *J. Hypertens.* 1996; 14: 355-63.
[51] Fu QG, Carstens E, Stelzer B, Zimmermann M. B vitamins suppress spinal dorsal horn nociceptive neurons in the cat. *Neurosci. Lett.* 1988; 95: 192-7.
[52] Zimmerman M, Bartoszyk GD, Bonke D, Jurna I, Wild A. Antinociceptive properties of pyridoxine. Neurophysiological and behavioral findings. *Ann. N Y Acad. Sci.* 1990; 585: 219-30.
[53] Bernstein AL, Dinesen JS. Brief communication: effect of pharmacologic doses of vitamin B6 on carpal tunnel syndrome, electroencephalographic results, and pain. *J. Am. Coll. Nutr.* 1993; 12: 73-6.
[54] Baldewicz T, Goodkin K, Feaster DJ, Blaney NT, Kumar M, Kumar A, Shor-Posner G, Baum M. Plasma pyridoxine deficiency is related to increased psychological distress in recently bereaved homosexual men. *Psychosom. Med.* 1998; 60: 297-308.
[55] McCarty MF. High-dose pyridoxine as an 'anti-stress' strategy. *Med. Hypotheses* 2000; 54: 803-7.

In: New Hope for Mental Disturbances
Editors: Vladimir Lerner and Chanoch Meodownik
ISBN 978-1-60692-691-8

Chapter 4

VITAMIN B_{12} AND FOLIC ACID IN COGNITIVE AND MENTAL DISORDERS

Yacov Grinshpun [1,3,4] ***and Tzvi Dwolatzky****[2,3,4]
1. Geriatric Department, Soroka Medical Center, Be'er Sheva, Israel
2. Geriatric Department, Mental Health Center, Be'er Sheva, Israel
3. Memory Clinic, Mental Health Center, Be'er Sheva, Israel
4. Faculty of Health Sciences, Ben Gurion University of the Negev, Be'er Sheva, Israel

INTRODUCTION

The initial clinical importance of folate and vitamin B12 (cobalamin) was related to their role in the development of macrocytic anemia. However, it subsequently became clear that these essential dietary substances played an important role in the functioning of the nervous system. Today there is increasing evidence that hematological and neuropsychiatric effects due to cobalamin and folate deficiency do not necessarily occur simultaneously. Mental or psychological changes may precede hematological signs by months or years, and they may in fact represent the initial or only symptoms.

The relationship between cobalamin and folate deficiency and psychiatric illness has been studied since these vitamins were first discovered in the 1940's. The mental effects described in the context of cobalamin deficiency cover a wide range of symptoms, varying from cognitive impairment (slow mentation, memory deficits, confusion, dementia), to mood changes (agitation, depression, mania) and even to psychotic episodes (paranoia, auditory and visual hallucinations, delusions). There is a clear association between folate and cognitive and mood disorders.

Evidence for direct effects of folate and cobalamin on brain functioning is compelling, and numerous associations of their deficiencies to mental illness are evident. The relationship

* Address for correspondence:*Tzvi Dwolatzky, Faculty of Health Sciences, Ben Gurion University of the Negev and Director, Department of Geriatrics and Memory Clinic, Be'er Sheva Mental Health Center. Mailing address: Be'er Sheva Mental Health Center, PO Box 4600, Be'er Sheva 84170, Israel. Tel: 08-6401520 Fax: 08-6401462. E-mail: tzvidov@bgu.ac.il.

of these vitamins to dementia is significant, but they are only rarely a cause of truly reversible dementia. These vitamin deficiencies may typically present initially with psychiatric symptoms, and physicians should thus be alert to the possibility of deficiencies of folate and cobalamin in various psychiatric populations. However, a direct causal relationship to specific neuropsychiatric illnesses has not yet been adequately elucidated. Further study is needed to refine our understanding of the method in which these vitamins contribute to conditions affecting cognitive and mental health.

In this chapter we will review historical perspectives relating to cobalamin and folate, we will discuss the physiology of these vitamins, and describe the clinical consequences of various neuropsychiatric deficiency syndromes.

HISTORY

The credit for developing the concept of vitamins is generally attributed to Kazimierz (Casimir) Funk, a polish biochemist, who described the “vital amines” or "vitamins" in 1912. His finding of a substance in brown rice (later termed vitamin B_1 or thiamine) was based on the discovery by Christiaan Eijkman that beri-beri was more common among those who ate fully-milled polished rice. The subsequent discovery and isolation of other vitamins transformed diseases, such as pellagra, scurvy and rickets, to curable conditions.

The history of folic acid and vitamin B_{12} is fascinating. The discovery of folic acid began in India in the 1920's where macrocytic (large cell) anemia of pregnancy was successfully treated by yeast and its proprietary extract "Marmite". Later, workers interested in poultry nutrition found that chicks grew slowly and developed a macrocytic anemia although they were fed on purified diets containing all of the known vitamins at that time. It was discovered in 1944 that this could be prevented by giving them crystalline "vitamin Bc" which had been isolated as a growth factor for certain bacteria. A similar closely related substance had also been obtained from spinach and named "folic acid" because of its origins from "foliage". The chemical structure of folic acid was identified in 1946 by Robert Stokstad.

It was known that foods containing animal protein were essential to prevent pernicious anemia (pernicious meaning "leading to death"). While it was recognized that sufferers of pernicious anemia lacked an "intrinsic factor" normally secreted by the stomach, the nature of the "extrinsic factor" that was present in meat, and in particular in liver, had not yet been identified. William P. Murphy, in delivering his lecture on receiving the Nobel Prize in Physiology or Medicine in 1934, described the dramatic clinical response that occurred when using injectable liver extract in treating pernicious anemia. This "liver factor" was finally isolated in 1948 and termed "vitamin B_{12}". The isolated crystals had a pink color, which was then found to result from the presence of cobalt, a trace metal. Thus this vitamin was also named "cobalamin".

The era of vitamin discovery flourished following this breakthrough, and although a number of other important substances have been detected since, this serves as a major foundation stone in the course of disease prevention by the provision of essential dietary nutrients. Cobalamin has an illustrious scientific history, culminating in the awarding of three Nobel Prizes relating to its discovery, its crystallographic characterization, and to the total synthesis of the compound.

PHYSIOLOGY

The metabolism of vitamin B_{12} (cobalamin) and folate is interrelated and both are necessary in several pathways in the central nervous system [1, 2]. Cobalamin and folate facilitate the production of S-adenosylmethionine (SAM) by promoting the conversion of homocysteine into methionine. In cases of folate or cobalamin deficiency methionine synthetase activity may be severely impaired, resulting in an elevated plasma total homocysteine level [3]. However, a high homocysteine level is not always related to vitamin deficiency [4]. Folate also influences the rate of synthesis of the neurotransmitters dopamine, norepinephrine, and serotonin, and acts as a cofactor in the hydroxylation of phenylalanine and tryptophan [5-7]. Disturbance of biogenic amine metabolism may lead to various psychiatric disorders.

Cobalamin and folate deficiency may contribute to the pathogenesis of neuropsychiatric disorders such as mental confusion, memory changes, cognitive slowing, mood disorder, violent behavior, fatigue, delirium, and paranoid psychosis. This relationship has been described by many investigators [6, 8-11]. Neuropsychiatric symptoms have been described as the presenting feature of cobalamin deficiency prior to the appearance of hematological findings [12, 13].

COBALAMIN

Physiology

Vitamin B_{12} or cyanocobalamin is a form of the cyanide-containing compounds known as cobalamins that is found in foods of animal origin, such as meat, shellfish, eggs and milk products. Cyanocobalamin is a complex cobalt-containing vitamin that is synthesized by microorganisms such as bacteria. Animals are not able to synthesize this compound since the enzymes required for its synthesis are not found in animals and plants.

Dietary vitamin B_{12} is bound either to haptocorrin, a 65-kDa glycoprotein produced by the salivary glands and gastrointestinal cells, or to intrinsic factor (a 49-kDa glycoprotein) secreted by the parietal cells in the gastric mucosa. Haptocorrin has a higher affinity for cyanocobalamin than does intrinsic factor, but since pancreatic proteases modify haptocorrin to a compound with less affinity, one may presume that effectively all cyanocobalamin reaches the small intestine bound to intrinsic factor. The intrinsic factor- cyanocobalamin complex then becomes bound to specific receptors in the ileum where it is absorbed by endocytosis. In the enterocytes, cyanocobalamin is transferred from intrinsic factor to transcobalamin II, another cyanocobalamin-binding protein that serves to transport it in the plasma.

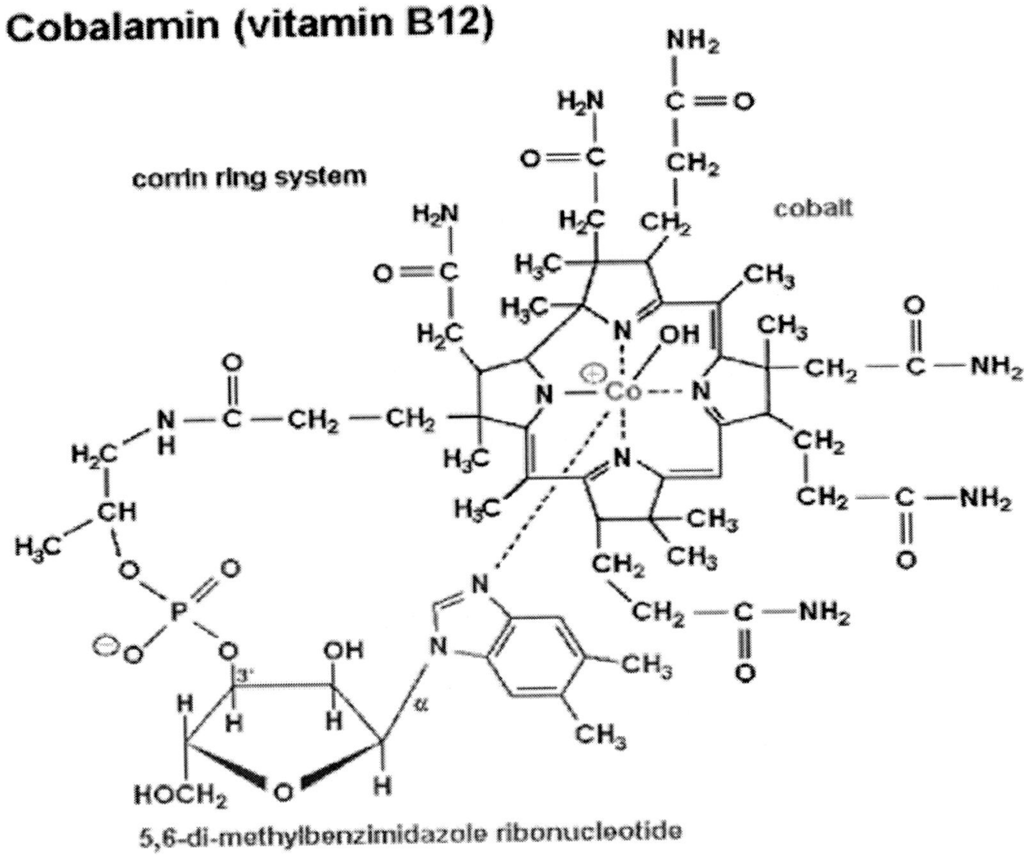

Vitamin B_{12} Deficiency

Deficiency due to an inadequate dietary intake of cyanocobalamin is very rare, and the clinical deficiency states are seen primarily in those cases where there is defective absorption of this vitamin. The daily requirement of vitamin B_{12}, which is found in most foods of animal origin, is 1-2 µg. The usual daily intake of B_{12} is between 5-7 µg and this is sufficient to supply daily requirements. This explains why dietary B_{12} deficiency occurs mainly in true vegans. With liver stores of between 2000-5000 µg and daily losses of B_{12} averaging 3-5 µg, clinical deficiency will develop more than 3 years following the cessation of absorption.

An inadequate production of intrinsic factor due to atrophic gastritis (pernicious anemia) is the most frequent cause of cobalamin deficiency. Bacterial overgrowth in the lumen of the intestine as a result of blind loop syndrome will compete with cobalamin. Gastrectomy, surgical resection of the terminal ileum and Crohn's disease are also important causes of cobalamin deficiency. Rarer causes are infections with fish tapeworm (Diphyllobothrium latum) pancreatic insufficiency and transcobalamin II deficiency.

Cobalamin deficiency presents most frequently with megaloblastic anemia. The anemia may be severe, with marked macrocytosis, leucopenia and thrombocytopenia. Changes in the mucosa lead to glossitis, anorexia or diarrhea. Neurologic changes affect peripheral nerves initially, with complaints of paresthesias, followed by involvement of the posterior columns resulting in abnormalities of gait and balance. Cognitive and neuropsychiatric changes follow, and these will be discussed in detail later in this chapter.

The true incidence of cerebral symptoms in cobalamin deficiency is unknown; with reports varying between 4% and almost 50%, depending on the population studied and on the definition of deficiency used. To date there is no universal agreement as to the "normal" range of serum vitamin B_{12} levels. A high incidence of hematologic, neurologic and gastrointestinal abnormalities in patients with serum vitamin B_{12} levels below 300 pg/ml lead investigators to conclude that the lower limit of normal should be between 300-350 pg/ml [14-16] and possibly even up to1000 pg/ml to maximize mental functioning [17]. Although some researchers have recommended an examination of serum methylmalonic acid (MMA) and/or homocysteine as a proof of cobalamin or folate deficiency [3], others conclude that increased plasma MMA and homocysteine are not pathognomonic markers and do not predict their clinical manifestations, stating that "those who suggest that serum MMA should replace serum cobalamin in assessing cobalamin status have not proved their case" [16].

FOLIC ACID

Physiology

Folic acid is the term commonly used for pteroylmonoglutamic acid, which, in its reduced form tetrahydrofolate, serves as an important mediator of one-carbon transfers. It is a water soluble vitamin found in most fruits and vegetables, particularly leafy green vegetables such as spinach, citrus fruits and dried peas and beans. It is also found in high concentrations in liver. Many processed foods, such as cereals, are supplemented with additional folate. A significant number of countries have adopted a universal policy of folate fortification of flour and standard bread products, in an effort to decrease the incidence of spina bifida in infants.

Folate is catalyzed to dihydrofolate and then to tetrahydrofolate by dihydrofolate reductase. The addition of methylene groups to tetrahydrofolate results in the formation of methylene tetrahydrofolate, which in turn is reduced to methyl tetrahydrofolate or oxidized to formyl tetrahydrofolate. Folate is an essential element in the production and maintenance of new cells and is required in DNA replication, where it plays an important role in the conversion of homocysteine to methionine and of deoxyuridalate to thymidylate.

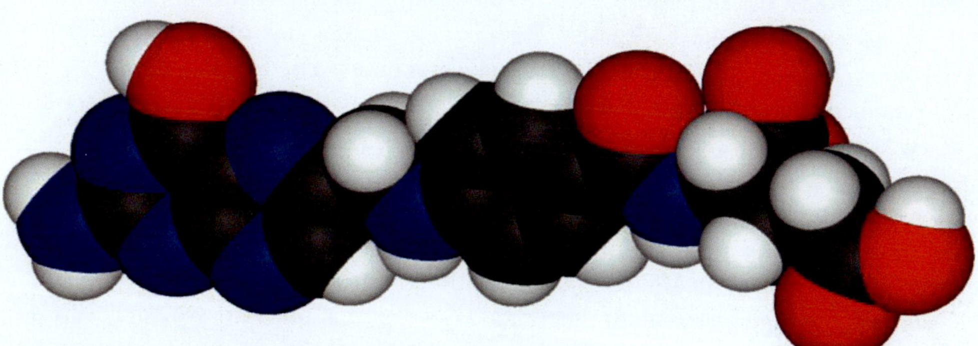

The structure of folic acid (from http://wikipedia.org).

Folate Deficiency

The recommended daily requirements of folate of 400 μg are usually supplied in the diet in developed countries, and the total body stores of about 5000 μg are sufficient to supply needs for 2 – 3 months. This having been said, a number of studies have found that most adults do not consume adequate amounts of folate when fortified foods are excluded from the calculation [18].

The most common cause of folate deficiency is dietary. This is found particularly in those patients who do not include fresh fruits and vegetables in their diet, such as alcoholics, patients with anorexia or food fetishes, or those with poor dentition such as the elderly with poorly fitting dentures who are unable to chew their food. Overcooking of vegetables will also decrease the availability of folate.

Decreased absorption of folate is seldom a cause of deficiency since the absorption of this substance occurs throughout the gastrointestinal tract. Tropical sprue may lead to folate deficiency. Absorption may be affected by drugs, such as sulfasalazine, phenytoin, and trimethoprim-sulfamethoxazole. Increased requirements for folate occur in pregnancy, chronic hemolytic anemia and exfoliative skin conditions. An increased loss of folate occurs in patients undergoing dialysis. The use of methotrexate is associated with a decrease in the reduction of folate to its active form.

In patients with increased requirements or who develop a folate deficiency, oral supplementation with 1mg/d is indicated. However, for those who are merely at risk, supplementation with a daily dose of 400 μg is sufficient. In fact, doses greater than 400 μg/day may be associated with a greater degree of cognitive decline over time [19].

Clinical folate deficiency presents with macrocytic anemia and changes in the mucosa. The anemia is of a megaloblastic type with macro-ovalocytes and hypersegmented neutrophils on peripheral blood smear. Serum folate deficiency is preferably determined according to the erythrocyte folate level, as this gives an indication of long-term folate status. The diagnosis of folate deficiency is confirmed by finding a red blood cell folate level of less than 150 ng/ml.

The Effect of Cobalamin and Folate on Cognition

An association between neuropsychiatric disorders and cobalamin deficiency has been recognized since 1849, when pernicious anemia was first described [20]. Cobalamin is an important cause of neurological disease, affecting the central nervous system (leading to impaired cognitive function), and the peripheral nervous system causing the syndrome of subacute combined degeneration of the spinal cord. These neural consequences of cobalamin deficiency are frequently irreversible.

In order to document the neurological consequences of cobalamin in a cohort of elderly patients with deficiency secondary to decreased absorption of the vitamin, some 92 patients were studied [21]. In this study cobalamin deficiency was defined as values less than 200 pg/ml. The most common neurologic manifestations were mild sensory polyneuropathy (44.6%), confusion or impaired mental functioning (22.8%) and physical asthenia (20.7%).

Folates are essential vitamins in the development of the central nervous system. The evidence for this association is clear, considering the causal relationship between low concentrations of folate at the time of conception and early pregnancy which may result in the development of congenital neural tube defects and syringomyelia [22]. Folate deficiency in adults is an important cause of megaloblastic anemia, and is associated with impaired cognitive function and dementing conditions such as Alzheimer's disease.

The relationship between cobalamin and folate on cognition has been well described in epidemiological studies. However, the exact physiological mechanism involved has yet to be determined, and many researchers still question whether the association between these substances and cognitive impairment in old age is causal or whether it is actually a consequence of disease [23].

Low serum levels of cobalamin and folate have been described in a large number of studies evaluating cognitive decline, particularly in older patients. A study evaluating the association between cognitive performance and plasma cobalamin, folate and homocysteine concentrations in the elderly among survivors of the Scottish Mental Surveys found these vitamins to be correlated with cognitive performance [24]. A cross-sectional community study investigated whether there was an association between homocysteine concentrations and cognitive impairment in an older African-Caribbean population. While a raised homocysteine level was significantly associated with cognitive impairment in this sample, it is important to note that this association was not explained by folate concentrations [25].

A small Greek study found that patients with dementia had significantly lower levels of folate and cobalamin than controls, and that higher plasma homocysteine levels were similarly associated with cognitive impairment [26]. In a larger study, 321 participants from the Veterans Affairs Normative Aging Study were subjected to cognitive assessment and levels of B-vitamins and homocysteine were measured [27]. Plasma homocysteine, folate, and vitamins B_6 and B_{12} were significantly associated with neuropsychological measures. Of interest in this study is that folate was protective against a decline in spatial copying ability over a 3-year period of follow-up. An Australian study evaluated the association between the dietary intake of cobalamin and folate, and self-reported cognitive function in 1183 middle-aged men and women [28]. A positive correlation was found between the levels of these vitamins and cognitive function. A study comparing the levels of homocysteine, folate and cobalamin in mild cognitive impairment (MCI), Alzheimer's disease and vascular dementia found that a low level of folate was associated with both MCI and dementia while hyperhomocysteinemia was associated with dementia [29]. Based on these findings they conclude that folate deficiency may precede the onset of dementia.

Other studies have failed to find a relationship between vitamin status and cognitive decline. A study of 75 patients in a long-term care setting in Ontario, Canada, found no significant difference between vitamin status and cognitive function [30]. The Leiden 85-Plus study assessed whether serum concentrations of homocysteine, cobalamin or folate predict cognitive decline in old age [23]. In this prospective, population-based, longitudinal study of almost 600 subjects aged 85 years who were followed up annually for four years, elevated serum concentrations of homocysteine and reduced folate levels were associated with cognitive impairment yet did not predict an increased rate of cognitive decline. It is important to note that in this study there was no association between the levels of cobalamin and cognitive function.

A rather interesting and unexpected finding was described by the authors of a large prospective study involving 3718 community-dwelling older persons in Chicago [19]. The rate of cognitive change over time was compared to the dietary intake of cobalamin and folate. While a high total cobalamin intake was associated with slower cognitive decline among the oldest participants, a high intake of folic acid was associated with a faster rate of cognitive decline. This finding raises important questions regarding the implications of high levels of dietary folate in older populations [19].

Vascular disease is important in the etiology of vascular dementia as well as Alzheimer's disease. In a study designed to evaluate the relationship between cobalamin/folate status and the presence of vascular disease in almost 2000 psychogeriatric patients, 7% of the study population had laboratory defined cobalamin/folate deficiencies. These deficiencies were rare in those patients younger than 70 years of age. There was also no association between Alzheimer's disease and cobalamin/folate deficiency, and the presence of vascular disease was higher among those patients with mild cognitive impairment (MCI) [31].

There is a growing body of literature studying the relationship between high levels of homocysteine, which is effected by folate and cobalamin, and cognitive function (see chapter on homocysteine). It is thus of significant interest to consider whether providing supplements of folate in the diet may improve or maintain cognitive function. It must be emphasized, however, that there is a risk in providing folate supplementation to those patients with anemia who have an undiagnosed cobalamin deficiency. Since both cobalamin and folate deficiencies causes an identical type of anemia, supplementation with folic acid alone in the presence of an associated cobalamin deficiency may correct the anemia but not prevent the progression of cobalamin associated neurological damage [20].

Much emphasis has been placed on identifying reversible causes of dementia, with the hope that treating these conditions will improve cognitive function and possibly prevent the devastating results of an otherwise progressive degenerative dementia. However, these potentially reversible dementias have been shown to occur less frequently than initially was thought to be the case and to respond poorly to treatment. In a 1988 meta-analysis of 32 studies, only 11% of almost 3000 patients "reversed" with 8% reversing partially and 3% fully [32]. The most common reversible or partially reversible causes of dementia were drug effects, depression, metabolic causes (such as cobalamin deficiency, hypercalcemia, thyroid or liver disease), normal pressure hydrocephalus, subdural hematomas, and tumors.

An updated meta-analysis by the same author found that while potentially reversible causes of dementia were seen in 9% of cases, only 0.6% actually reversed (0.29% partially and 0.31% fully) [33]. Although the dementia caused by these etiologies is in fact rarely reversible, these co-morbid conditions should nevertheless be sought and treated in their own right. There is limited evidence in the literature of reversible dementia due to cobalamin or folate deficiency. In fact, an evaluation of 560 incident cases of dementia in Rochester, Minnesota, found no patients to have cobalamin or folate deficiency [34].

In spite of the low yield, it remains accepted practice to routinely perform an evaluation of serum cobalamin and folate levels for those patients presenting with cognitive impairment and dementia, regardless of their age and previous state of health.

Vitamin B_{12} and Folate in Psychiatry

The relationship of cobalamin and folate deficiency to psychiatric illness has been studied and debated since these vitamins were first discovered in the 1940's. Cobalamin deficiency has been associated with many psychiatric illnesses and symptoms, and especially mood disorders, paranoid psychoses, violent behavior and fatigue. The clinical reviews, case reports and scientific basis of these conditions are the subject of much interest and research.

The reported prevalence of a low serum cobalamin level among psychiatric inpatients varies between 5% to 30% and that of a low serum folate level 10% to 33% [6, 7, 9, 35]. These findings are in contrast with a nonpsychiatric population in which only 3%-5% had low cobalamin levels and 5%-8% low folate levels [36-38]. Several studies have shown a higher incidence of cobalamin and folate deficiency in chronic psychiatric outpatients and inpatients [10, 14, 35, 39-41].

In a study comparing cobalamin and folate levels in newly admitted psychiatric patients to those of healthy controls, significantly lower levels of folate were found in the patient group (30% vs. 2.5%; $p<0.001$) [42]. Also, although cobalamin deficiency was common in these patients (26%), the control group had a similar degree of deficiency (25%). These findings of folate deficiency in patients suffering from mood disorders are consistent with those of other studies [6, 13, 43-48]. In patients with a depressed state the folate level was 3.5 times higher than those in a manic state [9, 46, 49, 50]. However, such a difference was not found with cobalamin.

Several studies have examined the serum levels of cobalamin and folate among newly admitted middle-aged psychiatric patients, and a relatively low prevalence of below normal levels of cobalamin was described (1% to 10%) [49, 51-53]. It has been reported that between 12%-30% of newly admitted patients with depression were found to have folate deficiency [13, 43-47, 54].

The increased prevalence of both cobalamin and folate deficiencies among newly admitted psychiatric patients are unlikely to result solely from alterations in the manifestation of mental illnesses, or by abnormal eating habits or dietary deficiencies. Vitamin deficiencies may play a role in the pathogenesis of psychiatric illnesses or lead to an exacerbation of preexisting mental disorders. Since the neuropsychiatric symptoms frequently appear before the hematological manifestations [7, 8], the clinical neuropsychiatric picture of cobalamin deficiency should not be based on hematological findings [55, 56].

It has been suggested that the evaluation of serum cobalamin and folate levels should be implemented routinely for all newly diagnosed psychiatric patients [11, 35, 39, 57]. Although these recommendations have not yet been widely accepted, studies certainly support the evaluation of folate levels in these patients. The association between cobalamin and/or folate deficiencies and mental (psychiatric) disturbances presents an important target for further research and clinical innovations. Larger studies are needed in order to further evaluate this relationship.

Summary

Cobalamin and folate are closely related vitamins involved in homocysteine metabolism. Epidemiologic studies have shown these compounds to be associated with neuropsychiatric conditions, including cognitive impairment and dementia, mood disorders and psychosis. Since normal hematological indices do not rule out deficiency, clinicians should remain vigilant to the possibility of deficiencies of folate and cobalamin in diverse psychiatric populations. The diagnosis and management of these deficiencies in this context remains a matter of debate. The quality of clinical investigation in this area is improving, but there are many unanswered questions that affect clinical practice. Ongoing research in this area will help to further elucidate these questions.

REFERENCES

[1] Shane B, Stokstad EL. Vitamin B12-folate interrelationships. *Annu. Rev. Nutr.* 1985; 5: 115-41.

[2] Chanarin I, Deacon R, Lumb M, Perry J. Cobalamin-folate interrelations. *Blood Rev.* 1989; 3: 211-5.

[3] Stabler SP, Marcell PD, Podell ER, Allen RH, Savage DG, Lindenbaum J. Elevation of total homocysteine in the serum of patients with cobalamin or folate deficiency detected by capillary gas chromatography-mass spectrometry. *J. Clin. Invest* 1988; 81: 466-74.

[4] Curtis D, Sparrow R, Brennan L, Van der Weyden MB. Elevated serum homocysteine as a predictor for vitamin B12 or folate deficiency. *Eur. J. Haematol.* 1994; 52: 227-32.

[5] Bottiglieri T, Hyland K, Laundy M, Godfrey P, Carney MW, Toone BK, Reynolds EH. Folate deficiency, biopterin and monoamine metabolism in depression. *Psychol. Med.* 1992; 22: 871-6.

[6] Bottiglieri T. Folate, vitamin B12, and neuropsychiatric disorders. *Nutr. Rev.* 1996; 54: 382-90.

[7] Hutto BR. Folate and cobalamin in psychiatric illness. *Compr. Psychiatry* 1997; 38: 305-14.

[8] Evans DL, Edelsohn GA, Golden RN. Organic psychosis without anemia or spinal cord symptoms in patients with vitamin B12 deficiency. *Am. J. Psychiatry* 1983; 140: 218-21.

[9] Hector M, Burton JR. What are the psychiatric manifestations of vitamin B12 deficiency?. *J. Am. Geriatr. Soc.* 1988; 36: 1105-12.

[10] Skerritt UM. A prevalence study of folate deficiency in a psychiatric in-patient population. *Acta Psychiatr. Scand.* 1998; 97: 228-32.

[11] Lerner V, Kanevsky M. Acute dementia with delirium due to vitamin B12 deficiency: a case report. *Int. J. Psychiatry Med.* 2002; 32: 215-20.

[12] Lindenbaum J, Healton EB, Savage DG, Brust JC, Garrett TJ, Podell ER, Marcell PD, Stabler SP, Allen RH. Neuropsychiatric disorders caused by cobalamin deficiency in the absence of anemia or macrocytosis. *N Engl. J. Med.* 1988; 318: 1720-8.

[13] Godfrey PS, Toone BK, Carney MW, Flynn TG, Bottiglieri T, Laundy M, Chanarin I, Reynolds EH. Enhancement of recovery from psychiatric illness by methylfolate. *Lancet* 1990; 336: 392-5.

[14] Yao Y, Yao SL, Yao SS, Yao G, Lou W. Prevalence of vitamin B12 deficiency among geriatric outpatients. *J. Fam. Pract.* 1992; 35: 524-8.

[15] Swain R. An update of vitamin B12 metabolism and deficiency states. *J. Fam. Pract.* 1995; 41: 595-600.

[16] Chanarin I, Metz J. Diagnosis of cobalamin deficiency: the old and the new. *Br. J. Haematol.* 1997; 97: 695-700.

[17] Dommisse J. Subtle vitamin-B12 deficiency and psychiatry: a largely unnoticed but devastating relationship? *Med. Hypotheses* 1991; 34: 131-40.

[18] Raiten DJ, Fisher KD. Assessment of folate methodology used in the Third National Health and Nutrition Examination Survey (NHANES III, 1988-1994). *J. Nutr.* 1995; 125: 1371S-1398S.

[19] Morris MC, Evans DA, Bienias JL, Tangney CC, Hebert LE, Scherr PA, Schneider JA. Dietary folate and vitamin B12 intake and cognitive decline among community-dwelling older persons. *Arch Neurol.* 2005; 62: 641-5.

[20] Malouf R, Areosa Sastre A. Vitamin B12 for cognition. *Cochrane Database Syst. Rev.* 2003: CD004326.

[21] Andres E, Affenberger S, Vinzio S, Kurtz JE, Noel E, Kaltenbach G, Maloisel F, Schlienger JL, Blickle JF. Food-cobalamin malabsorption in elderly patients: clinical manifestations and treatment. *Am. J. Med.* 2005; 118: 1154-9.

[22] Vieira AR, Murray JC, Trembath D, Orioli IM, Castilla EE, Cooper ME, Marazita ML, Lennon-Graham F, Speer M. Studies of reduced folate carrier 1 (RFC1) A80G and 5,10-methylenetetrahydrofolate reductase (MTHFR) C677T polymorphisms with neural tube and orofacial cleft defects. *Am. J. Med. Genet.* A 2005; 135: 220-3.

[23] Mooijaart SP, Gussekloo J, Frolich M, Jolles J, Stott DJ, Westendorp RG, de Craen AJ. Homocysteine, vitamin B-12, and folic acid and the risk of cognitive decline in old age: the Leiden 85-Plus study. Am. J. Clin. Nutr. *2005; 82: 866-71.*

[24] *Duthie SJ, Whalley LJ,* Collins AR, Leaper S, Berger K, Deary IJ. Homocysteine, B vitamin status, and cognitive function in the elderly. *Am. J. Clin. Nutr.* 2002; 75: 908-13.

[25] Stewart R, Asonganyi B, Sherwood R. Plasma homocysteine and cognitive impairment in an older British African-Caribbean population. *J. Am. Geriatr. Soc.* 2002; 50: 1227-32.

[26] Dimopoulos N, Piperi C, Salonicioti A, Psarra V, Gazi F, Nounopoulos C, Lea RW, Kalofoutis A. Association of cognitive impairment with plasma levels of folate, vitamin B12 and homocysteine in the elderly. *In Vivo* 2006; 20: 895-9.

[27] Tucker KL, Qiao N, Scott T, Rosenberg I, Spiro A, 3rd. High homocysteine and low B vitamins predict cognitive decline in aging men: the Veterans Affairs Normative Aging Study. *Am. J. Clin. Nutr.* 2005; 82: 627-35.

[28] Bryan J, Calvaresi E. Associations between dietary intake of folate and vitamins B-12 and B-6 and self-reported cognitive function and psychological well-being in Australian men and women in midlife. *J. Nutr. Health Aging* 2004; 8: 226-32.

[29] Quadri P, Fragiacomo C, Pezzati R, Zanda E, Forloni G, Tettamanti M, Lucca U. Homocysteine, folate, and vitamin B-12 in mild cognitive impairment, Alzheimer disease, and vascular dementia. *Am. J. Clin. Nutr.* 2004; 80: 114-22.

[30] Paulionis L, Kane SL, Meckling KA. Vitamin status and cognitive function in a long-term care population. *BMC Geriatr.* 2005; 5: 16.

[31] Nilsson K, Gustafson L, Hultberg B. Plasma homocysteine, cobalamin/folate status, and vascular disease in a large population of psychogeriatric patients. *Dement Geriatr. Cogn. Disord.* 2006; 22: 358-66.

[32] Clarfield AM. The reversible dementias: do they reverse? *Ann. Intern. Med.* 1988; 109: 476-86.

[33] Clarfield AM. The decreasing prevalence of reversible dementias: an updated meta-analysis. *Arch Intern. Med.* 2003; 163: 2219-29.

[34] Knopman DS, Petersen RC, Cha RH, Edland SD, Rocca WA. Incidence and causes of nondegenerative nonvascular dementia: a population-based study. *Arch Neurol.* 2006; 63: 218-21.

[35] Silver H. Vitamin B12 levels are low in hospitalized psychiatric patients. *Isr. J. Psychiatry Relat. Sci.* 2000; 37: 41-5.

[36] Garry PJ, Goodwin JS, Hunt WC. Folate and vitamin B12 status in a healthy elderly population. *J. Am. Geriatr. Soc.* 1984; 32: 719-26.

[37] Grinblat J, Marcus DL, Hernandez F, Freedman ML. Folate and vitamin B12 levels in an urban elderly population with chronic diseases. Assessment of two laboratory folate assays: microbiologic and radioassay. *J. Am. Geriatr. Soc.* 1986; 34: 627-32.

[38] de Carvalho MJ, Guilland JC, Moreau D, Boggio V, Fuchs F. Vitamin status of healthy subjects in Burgundy (France). *Ann. Nutr. Metab.* 1996; 40: 24-51.

[39] Teunisse S, Bollen AE, van Gool WA, Walstra GJ. Dementia and subnormal levels of vitamin B12: effects of replacement therapy on dementia. *J. Neurol.* 1996; 243: 522-9.

[40] Greer A, McBride DH, Shenkin A. Comparison of the nutritional state of new and long-term patients in a psychogeriatric unit. *Br. J. Psychiatry* 1986; 149: 738-41.

[41] Bell IR, Edman JS, Marby DW, Satlin A, Dreier T, Liptzin B, Cole JO. Vitamin B12 and folate status in acute geropsychiatric inpatients: affective and cognitive characteristics of a vitamin nondeficient population. *Biol. Psychiatry* 1990; 27: 125-37.

[42] Lerner V, Kanevsky M, Dwolatzky T, Rouach T, Kamin R, Miodownik C. Vitamin B12 and folate serum levels in newly admitted psychiatric patients. *Clin. Nutr.* 2006; 25: 60-7.

[43] Alpert JE, Fava M. Nutrition and depression: the role of folate. Nutr Rev 1997; 55: 145-9.

[44] Alpert JE, Mischoulon D, Nierenberg AA, Fava M. Nutrition and depression: focus on folate. *Nutrition* 2000; 16: 544-6.

[45] Bjelland I, Ueland PM, Vollset SE. Folate and depression. *Psychother. Psychosom.* 2003; 72: 59-60.

[46] Carney MW, Chary TK, Laundy M, Bottiglieri T, Chanarin I, Reynolds EH, Toone B. Red cell folate concentrations in psychiatric patients. *J. Affect Disord.* 1990; 19: 207-13.

[47] Morris MS, Fava M, Jacques PF, Selhub J, Rosenberg IH. Depression and folate status in the US Population. *Psychother. Psychosom.* 2003; 72: 80-7.

[48] Reynolds EH. Folic acid, ageing, depression, and dementia. *Bmj* 2002; 324: 1512-5.

[49] Carney MW. Serum folate values in 423 psychiatric patients. *BMJ* 1967; 4: 512-6.

[50] Tiemeier H, van Tuijl HR, Hofman A, Meijer J, Kiliaan AJ, Breteler MM. Vitamin B12, folate, and homocysteine in depression: the Rotterdam Study. *Am. J. Psychiatry* 2002; 159: 2099-101.

[51] Edwin E, Holten K, Norum K, et al. Vitamin B12 hypovitaminosis in mental dieases [letter]. *Acta Med. Scand.* 1965; 177: 689.

[52] Elsborg L, Hansen T, Rafaelsen OJ. Vitamin B12 concentrations in psychiatric patients. *Acta Psychiatr. Scand.* 1979; 59: 145-52.

[53] Hansen T, Rafaelson O, Rodbro P. Vitamin B12 deficiency in psychiatry. *Lancet* 1966; 2: 965.

[54] McLaughlin B, McMahon A. Folate and depression. *Br. J. Psychiatry* 1993; 162: 572.
[55] Goodman M, Chen XH, Darwish D. Are U.S. lower normal B12 limits too low? *J. Am. Geriatr. Soc.* 1996; 44: 1274-5.
[56] Green R, Kinsella LJ. Current concepts in the diagnosis of cobalamin deficiency. *Neurology* 1995; 45: 1435-40.
[57] Fava M, Borus JS, Alpert JE, Nierenberg AA, Rosenbaum JF, Bottiglieri T. Folate, vitamin B12, and homocysteine in major depressive disorder. *Am. J. Psychiatry* 1997; 154: 426-8.

In: New Hope for Mental Disturbances
Editors: Vladimir Lerner and Chanoch Meodownik
ISBN 978-1-60692-691-8

Chapter 5

HOMOCYSTEINE AS A RISK FACTOR IN SCHIZOPHRENIA

Joseph Levine[1]***, Anna Bromberg and Tzvi Dwolatzky***
Division of Psychiatry, Ministry of Health Be'er Sheva Mental Health Center,
Faculty of Health Sciences Ben-Gurion University of the Negev, Be'er-Sheva, Israel

ABSTRACT

Homocysteine (Hcy) is an amino acid generated via methionine metabolism suggested to be rapidly taken up by neurons via a specific membrane transporter. Several enzymes, including methylenetetrahydrofolate reductase, methionine synthase and cystathionine beta-synthase, are involved in homocysteine metabolism and vitamins B_{12} and B_6 and folate serve as co-factors for these and other enzymes involved in homocysteine metabolism.

Homocysteine is suggested to be a neurotoxic amino acid via its effects on the NMDA receptors and/or the cell redox status.

Elevated plasma homocysteine has been found to be a risk factor for Alzheimer's disease as well as cerebral vascular disease, suggesting that some risk factors can accelerate or increase the severity of several CNS disease processes.

We screened 193 chronic schizophrenic patients from our region for plasma homocysteine levels and compared them with 762 controls (evaluated in a screening program for employee health). Mean homocysteine level was 16.3 ± 11.8 (SD) μM in schizophrenic patients vs. 10.6 ± 3.6 (SD) μM in healthy controls. The elevation in homocysteine was statistically significant and was evident almost entirely in young male schizophrenic patients. A second study in 184 consecutively admitted schizophrenic patients and 305 control subjects showed similar results.

Homocysteine can be lowered by providing oral folic acid, vitamin B_{12} and pyridoxine. Forty-two schizophrenic patients with plasma homocysteine levels above 15 μM were treated either with these vitamins for three months or placebo for three months

[1] Corresponding author: Joseph Levine, Faculty of Health Sciences, Ben Gurion University of the Negev and Psychiatric Department at Be'er Sheva Mental Health Center. Mail address: Be'er Sheva Mental Health Center, PO Box 4600, Be'er Sheva 84170, Israel, Tel.: +972-8-6401401; Fax: +972-8-6401621; Email: yossilevine@gmail.com.

in a randomized double-blind placebo controlled crossover design. Homocysteine levels significantly declined on vitamin therapy compared to placebo in all patients except for one non-compliant subject. Clinical symptoms of schizophrenia as measured by the Positive and Negative Syndrome Scale (PANSS) declined significantly more in those on active treatment compared with placebo. Of the neuropsychological test results, the Wisconsin Card Sort (Categories Completed) results were significantly better after vitamin treatment than after placebo.

A subgroup of schizophrenic patients with hyperhomocysteinemia may thus benefit from the addition of B vitamins, a fairly simple therapeutic strategy.

Homocysteine May Consist A Risk Factor For Schizophrenia

Homocysteine (Hcy) is an amino acid generated via methionine metabolism [1] and suggested to be rapidly taken up by neurons via a specific membrane transporter [2]. Several enzymes, including methylenetetrahydrofolate reductase, methionine synthase and cystathionine beta-synthase are involved in homocysteine metrabolism, and vitamins B_{12} and B_6 and folate serve as co-factors for these and other enzymes involved in homocysteine metabolism.

The methyl donor in most methylation reactions is S-adenosylmethionine (SAM), produced from the dietary amino acid methionine. After the donation of the methyl group, SAM is converted to S-adenosylhomocysteine (SAH). Under normal conditions SAH is rapidly hydrolyzed to homocysteine. SAH inhibits the activity of most SAM-dependent methyltransferases [3]. A high intracellular homocysteine level shifts the equilibrium between SAH and homocysteine back to SAH production [3] and causes global hypomethylation [4]. See figure 1 below.

Methionine loading is known to increase plasma homocysteine levels. Interestingly, more than 30 years ago Antun et al [5] following Pollin et al [6] reported that 10-20g of L-methionine orally may exacerbate psychosis in chronic schizophrenic patients [7].

Regland et al. reported a case of a young schizophrenic patient with a significantly increased serum level of homocysteine [8]. She improved each time that she was treated with cobalamin (B_{12}) injections and deteriorated in periods without treatment.

Following the above case report, Regland et al. evaluated patients with schizophrenia-like psychosis [9]. Seven of 11 patients, six males and one female, were homozygous for thermolabile methylenetetrahydrofolate reductase (MTHFR), a variant of the enzymes demonstrating reduced activity that may lead to an increased homocysteine plasma level. In the patients who were homozygous for the C677T mutation, the homocysteine concentrations did not respond to vitamin B_{12} but were normalized by folate supplementation. These authors suggested that homozygosity for thermolabile MTHFR is a risk factor for schizophrenia-like psychosis and that this risk may be reduced by folate supplementation.

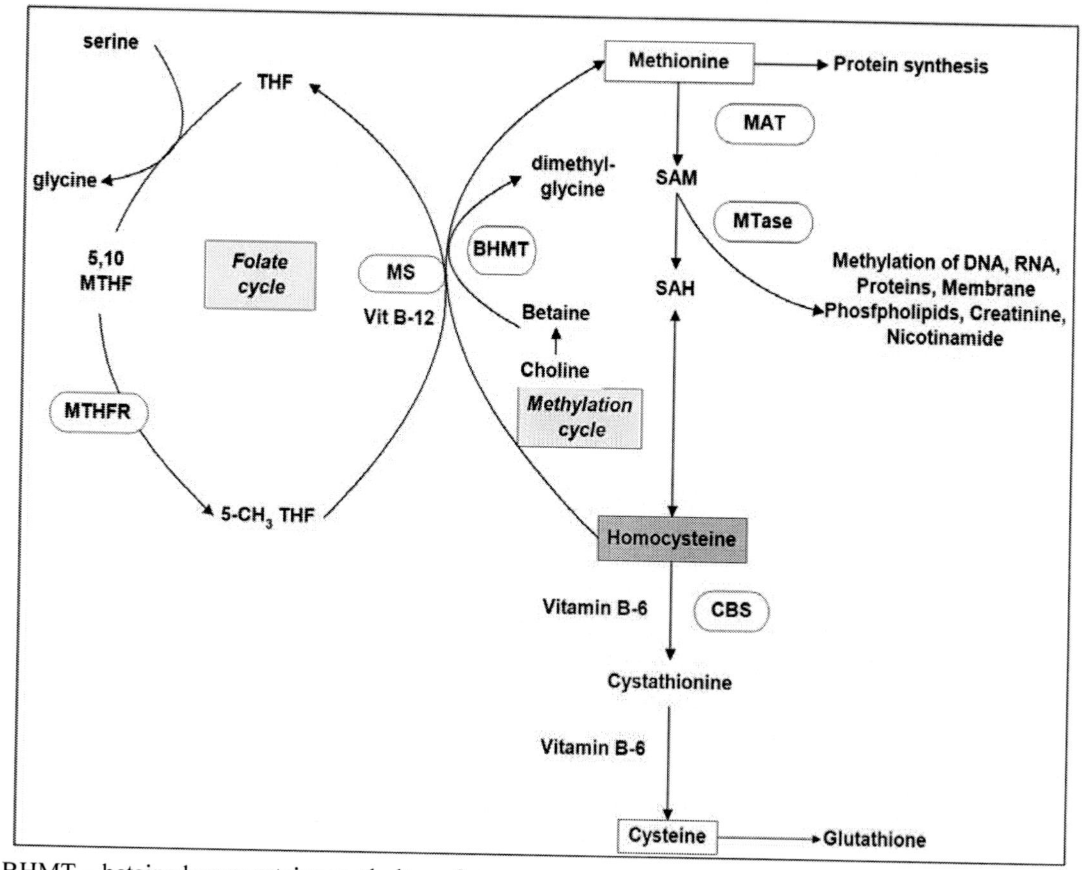

BHMT – betaine homocysteine methyltransferase.
MAT – methionine adenosyltransferase.
DHF – dehyrofolate.
MTase – methyltransferase.
MTHFR – methyltetrahydrofolate reductase.
CBS – cystathionine synthase.
THF – tetrohydrofolate.
5-CH_3 THF methyltetrahydrofolate.
5,10 MTHF – 5,10 dimethyltetrahydrofolate.
SAM – *S*-adenosylmethionine.
SAH – *S*-adenosylhomocysteine.

Figure 1. Homocysteine Metabolic Pathways.

Susser et al. conducted a pilot study comparing homocysteine levels of schizophrenic patients and normal controls with and without low folate levels [10]. In the low folate group (6 cases, 8 controls), mean homocysteine was 10.7 μM in schizophrenic patients compared with 7.7 μM in controls (p = .03), whereas in the non-low folate group (11 cases, 16 controls) mean homocysteine did not differ between schizophrenic patients and controls. These pilot data support the hypothesis that a folate-sensitive defect in homocysteine metabolism may contribute to schizophrenia in some individuals.

The origin of elevated plasma homocysteine in schizophrenia is unclear, but epidemiological studies suggest that poor nutrition, smoking, lack of exercise and obesity can contribute to elevated homocysteine levels [11].

As suggested above a common genetic polymorphism of MTHFR may also predispose individuals to elevated homocysteine [12] especially in the presence of epidemiological risk factors. However, although there are more studies that seem to support the association between polymorphism and schizophrenia, this opinion is not universal (see studies, meta-analyses and reviews [13-29]).

We have screened for plasma homocysteine levels in schizophrenic patients and compared the results with those of a control population [30].

One hundred and ninety-three chronic schizophrenic patients (with a diagnosis of this condition based on DSM-IV criteria), including males and females aged 18-70 years, with no history of neurologic or cardiovascular disorders or drug and alcohol abuse, agreed to participate in the study. All were drug-treated and were in a variety of clinical settings, including acute inpatient units, chronic inpatient units, community hostels and outpatient care.

Controls were males and females between the ages of 18-70 years who were randomly selected from employee health screening programs, which included the determination of plasma homocysteine levels. Laboratory testing was performed in both groups over the same time period of time.

Morning fasting blood samples were obtained in ice-cooled EDTA (ethylenediaminetetraacetic acid) tubes. Plasma was separated by centrifugation at 5°C and stored at -20°C. Total homocysteine levels were measured by HPLC technology with fluorescence detection following labeling of homocysteine with monobromobimane as a modification of the method of Araki and Sako [31].

A one-way ANOVA with age and sex as covariants was performed. The effect of schizophrenia was marked ($F=136$, $df= 1;951$, $p<0.0001$) and mean homocysteine level was $16.4 \pm 12\mu M$ (SD) in schizophrenic patients vs. $10.6 \pm 4\mu M$ (SD) in healthy controls. The elevation in homocysteine was statistically significant and was evident almost entirely in male schizophrenic patients younger than 50 years of age. Plasma vitamin B_{12} and folic acid demonstrated an inverse correlation with plasma homocysteine, but this did not explain the majority of the variance (see [33] for more details).

Following the finding of high homocysteine levels in patients with schizophrenia [30], our group conducted another study in which newly admitted schizophrenic patients to the Be'er Sheva Mental Health Center were screened for serum homocysteine [32]. Patients with physical illnesses, including neurological, hepatic, renal, endocrine (including diabetes) or cardiovascular diseases, or those with alcohol or drug abuse in the previous 6 months, were excluded.

The serum homocysteine was analyzed by means of three-way ANOVA by age, sex and diagnosis. There was a significant effect of diagnosis ($F= 16$, $df= 1,473$, $p<0.001$) and sex ($F=14$, $df= 1,473$, $p<0.001$) but no significant effect of age. There was a significant interaction between sex and diagnosis ($F=8.3$, $df= 1,473$, $p<0.005$). Here as well the increase in homocysteine was found entirely in male schizophrenic patients below the age of 50 years. Mean $\pm$ S.D. homocysteine level (μM) are summarized in Table 1:

Table 1. Homocysteine Levels In Newly Admitted Schizophrenia Patients And Healthy Controls (Modified From Applebaum Et Al. [32])

Schizophrenia patients (n=184)			Control subjects (n=305)	
Age(years)	Men (n=127)	Women (n=57)	Men (n=151)	Women (n=154)
20-30	18.2 ±16 (n=36)*	11.1±2.9 (n=18)	8.3±2 (n=29)	9.2±2.0(n=36)
31-40	13.7±5 (n=36) *	11.2±3.2 (n=15)	10.5±2 (n=32)	9.9±2.5 (n=31)
41-50	14.1±6 (n=36) *	10.4±4.0 (n=16)	11.6±2 (n=35)	10.7±2.4 (n=30)
51-70	12.8±4.3 (n=19)	11.7±2.8 (n=8)	13.3±2 (n=55)	12.1±2.0 (n=57)

* Statistical difference from the corresponding control group (ANOVA, p<0.05).

The finding that young newly admitted schizophrenia patients have a similarly elevated blood homocysteine as reported previously in a group consisting of mainly institutionalized schizophrenic patients suggests that this increase is probably not related to an institutional diet. Nevertheless, it is certainly possible that patients in the weeks or months prior to admission may be subject to poor nutrition even at home. As stated previously, the finding by Levine et al [30] that plasma vitamin B_{12} and folic acid demonstrated an inverse correlation with plasma homocysteine did not explain a majority of the variance [33]. There seems to be an increased rate of smoking among schizophrenic male patients compared with controls. Smoking may raise homocysteine by 1-2 μM [34] but this effect is not large enough to explain our findings.

Our results are confirmed by a recent meta-analysis by Muntjewerff et al of eight retrospective studies (812 cases and 2113 control subjects) which examined the association between homocysteine and schizophrenia, with the authors reporting that a 5 micromol/l higher homocysteine level was associated with a 70% higher risk of schizophrenia [29].

It is of note that a recent report suggests that an elevated homocysteine level may also appear in male adolescents with schizophrenia [35]. The authors conducted a prospective case-control study, comparing plasma homocysteine levels in a group of adolescents with schizophrenia to normal healthy controls. Mean plasma homocysteine levels were significantly higher in the patient group than in the control group (15.4±2.0 versus 9.8±0.3 μM, respectively, p<0.03). The difference was almost entirely attributable to the adolescent male schizophrenia subgroup.

What Are the Proposed Mechanisms of Homocysteine Neurotoxicity in Schizophrenia?

A. Elevated Homocysteine in Schizophrenia May Lead to Altered N-methyl-D-aspartate Glutamatergic Receptor Activity

N-methyl-D-aspartate (NMDA) receptors are closely regulated by a number of regulatory sites, including the glycine co-agonist site that is necessary for the receptor activation.

In general, homocysteine affects NMDA glutamatergic systems [36-38] and these systems are reported to play some role in the pathogenesis of schizophrenia.

Lipton et al suggested that the neurotoxicity of homocysteine may be associated with the dual actions of homocysteine at the N-methyl-D-aspartate receptor [37].

Under normal conditions CSF glycine levels are much lower than that of the plasma and are suggested to be 10-1 μM versus 150-200 μM respectively [39]. Under these normal conditions, it is suggested that homocysteine acts as an NMDA receptor antagonist at the glycine site and causes NMDA receptor hypofunction. It is of note that NMDA receptor hypofunction is implicated in the etiology of schizophrenia [40] and that patients with schizophrenia are reported to exhibit low plasma glycine levels and glycine-serine ratios along with elevated homocysteine levels compared with controls [41]. It is thus suggested that in schizophrenic patients with relatively intact blood brain barrier (BBB) (preventing the entrance of peripheral glycine into the brain extracellular fluids), the presence of a mild elevation of homocysteine levels may further enhance such NMDA receptor hypofunction.

However, homocysteine can also act as a NMDA receptor agonist at glutamate sites when the glycine levels in the brain extracellular fluids (as reflected by CSF glycine level) are higher than normal and close to the levels in the plasma [37] leading to the overstimulation of N-methyl-D-aspartate receptors. In general, this situation has been suggested to occur in the presence of head trauma and stroke, where the integrity of the BBB is impaired [39, 42]. Under such conditions homocysteine is neurotoxic via its agonistic action on the N-methyl-D-Aspartate (NMDA) receptor.

In normal circumstances, the NMDA receptor is activated endogenously by the excitatory amino acid glutamate and its activation increases intracellular Ca^{2+} concentration. In case of overstimulation the enhanced increase intracellular Ca^{2+} concentration may be followed by the release of cellular proteases and cell death [37, 43, 44]. This mechanism of cell death is called excitotoxicity and is implicated in a wide variety of neurodegenerative conditions and may be involved in the neurodegenerative alterations reported in schizophrenia. In this regard some authors have suggested a link between apopotic processes and schizophrenia [45, 46].

Interestingly, high homocysteine levels may lead to impairment of BBB integrity [47]. In this regard, plasma homocysteine concentrations of approximately 30-98μM in mice (being an increase of 7-20 fold above normal levels) led to impairment of BBB integrity [47, 48]. Stress as well is suggested to be involved in impairment to the BBB [49, 50]. Stress may also be associated with elevated homocysteine levels [51].

We propose that in schizophrenic patients with mild elevation of homocysteine levels and a clinically stable condition (hypothesized not to be associated with increased stress), the BBB will be intact, whereas in schizophrenic patients with mild elevation of homocysteine levels in an unstabilized phase of their illness (hypothesized to be characterized by considerable stress), the integrity of the BBB will be impaired leading to increased CNS glycine levels and possibly also to increased homocysteine levels in the brain extracellular fluid (homocysteine CSF levels are reported to be much lower than those in the plasma and impaired BBB function is thus suggested to result in increased homocysteine levels in the brain extracellular fluids) resulting in overstimulation of NMDA receptors and cell death.

We also propose that where homocysteine levels are moderately high, the integrity of the BBB may be impaired in spite of the fact that there is no increased stress. Such moderately high levels seem to appear in less then 5% of male patients with schizophrenia as supported by our data [30, 32]. In this circumstance we suggest that the hyperactivation of NMDA receptors may occur even in the stabilized phase of the illness which is theoretically not characterized by increased stress.

Figure 2 portrays the suggested dual effects of mild elevation of homocysteine on NMDA receptors

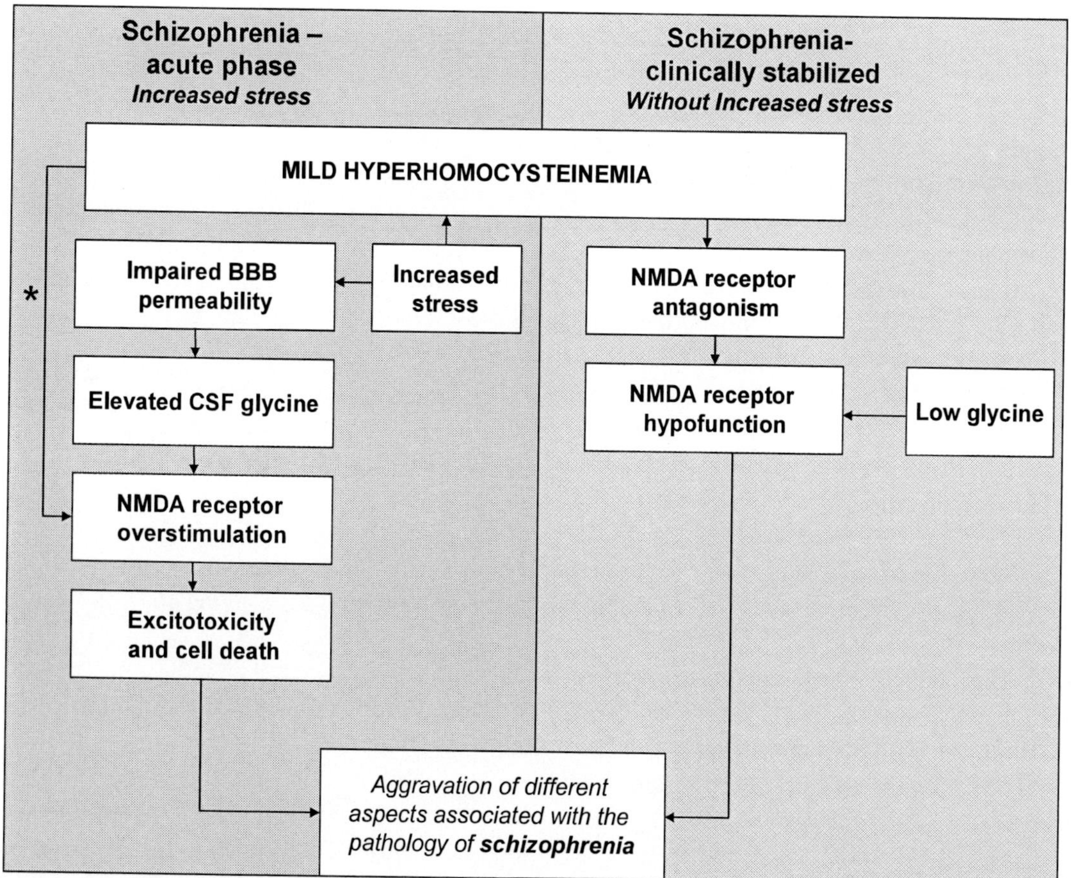

* Homocysteine may lead to activation of NMDA receptors in the face of elevated glycine in brain extracellular fluid.

Figure 2. hypothesized dual effects of mild elevatation of homocysteine on pathophysiology of schizophrenia via NMDA receptors.

B. Elevated Homocysteine in Schizophrenia may Lead to Enhanced Oxidative Stress

Oxidative damage inflicted by reactive oxygen species is also referred to as oxidative stress. Oxidative stress is the result of the increased formation of free radicals and reduced antioxidative processes. In other words, oxidative stress is a state of imbalance between the generation of reactive oxygen species and the antioxidant defense capacity of the body. It is suggested that neurons are especially sensitive to damage inflicted by free radicals and that this may result in the degeneration of neurons. This mechanism of neuronal degeneration was suggested in a variety of neurodegenerative diseases, including schizophrenia, and may be involved in the neurodegenerative alterations and cognitive impairments reported in this disorder as well as in its symptomatology (i.e, negative symptoms).

Increased homocysteine concentration is suggested to enhance the oxidative stress processes [36, 52, 53] and some propose that schizophrenia is characterized by an abnormal oxidative stress load. This is based on evidence of deregulation of free radical metabolism, as detected by abnormal activity of critical antioxidant enzymes as well as by findings that the gene of the key gluthatione-synthesizing enzyme, glutamate cysteine ligase modifier (GCLM) subunit, is strongly associated with schizophrenia [54-57]. In this regard psychosis score and negative symptoms have been associated with low levels of glutathione peroxidase [58]. Fendri et al and Nishioka et al have presented evidence for oxidative DNA damage and coordinated cell-cycle activation in elderly "poor-outcome" schizophrenia [56, 59].

It may thus be hypothesized that homocysteine may aggravate damage to brain tissue reported in schizophrenia and perhaps be related to some of its clinical manifestations by enhancing oxidative stress processes.

C. Elevated Homocysteine in Schizophrenia may Lead to DNA Hypomethylation

DNA methylation status is a dynamic feature and responds to different physiological and pathological conditions such as development, cell differentiation [60], aging [61] and cancer [62].

The methyl donor in most methylation reactions is S-adenosylmethionine (SAM), produced from the dietary amino acid methionine (see graph 1). After the donation of the methyl group SAM is converted to S-adenosylhomocysteine (SAH). Under normal conditions SAH is rapidly hydrolyzed to homocysteine. SAH inhibits the activity of most SAM-dependent methyltransferases [3]. High intracellular homocysteine level shifts the equilibrium between SAH and homocysteine back to SAH production [3]. Elevation of S-adenosyl-homocysteine was suggested to be associated with DNA hypomethylation and alterations in gene expression [4, 63].

MTHFR is considered to be one of the key enzymes in *de novo* SAM synthesis (Fig 1). The 677T allele of the MTHFR gene has been suggested to be associated both with elevated levels of homocysteine [64] and with neuropsychiatric disorders such as schizophrenia [9]. Recently, this allele was found to be significantly associated with global DNA hypomethylation [65, 66] and thus elevated homocysteine levels in schizophrenia may be associated with DNA hypomethylation, the latter possibly contributing to the pathogenesis of this illness. S-adenosyl-homocysteine is also a non-competitive inhibitor of catechol-O-methyltransferase (COMT). The more active allele of COMT is reported to be associated with schizophrenia [67] and although counterintuitive it might be that homocysteine may play some aggravating role in the pathogenesis of this illness through an indirect effect on COMT.

D. Elevated Homocysteine in Schizophrenia may Lead to Brain Neurodegeneration

Elevated plasma homocysteine could contribute to cognitive deterioration and cerebral atrophy [68, 69] and Bleich et al showed a significant positive relationship between plasma homocysteine levels and brain atrophy [70]. The mechanisms involved may be associated with those portrayed above or may yet to be determined. Such atrophic changes seem to be marked in young male – but not female - schizophrenia patients and this same group of young males with schizophrenia is reported to exhibit elevated homocysteine levels [30, 32]. Possible explanation for such a sex difference may include the protective effect of estrogen that may exert a protective effect in young females against the neurodegenerative processes associated with schizophrenia [71] similarly to its suggested role in the prevention of the neurodegenerative disease of Alzheimer's [72]. Such effect of estrogen may be mediated via its homocysteine lowering effect [52].

A Treatment Trial of Homocysteine Reducing Strategy in Schizophrenia Patients With Hyperhomocysteinemia

Folic acid, vitamin B_{12} and pyridoxine have marked homocysteine-reducing properties [73] and are under intensive study as possible preventive agents in cardiovascular disease, stroke and Alzheimer's disease.

Godfrey et al. reported that 6 months of folate administration as an adjunct to pharmacotherapy in schizophrenic patients demonstrating a borderline or deficient plasma folate level led to a symptomatic improvement that progresses with the length of treatment [74].

We therefore performed a study of these vitamins in schizophrenia patients selected for elevated plasma homocysteine levels [75].

Chronic schizophrenia patients were screened for plasma homocysteine [30, 32]. Patients with levels over 15 μM (the standard upper limit of plasma homocysteine in clinical laboratories) who had been continuously ill for at least one year were included after obtaining written informed consent. Patients with physical illness or an abnormality on blood chemistry or with alcohol or drug abuse were excluded. The design was a double-blind crossover study where patients received one tablet a day containing 2 mg folic acid, 25 mg pyridoxine and 400 μg B_{12}. After 3 months patients entered a crossover phase where those receiving active vitamin now received placebo and vice versa (see figure 3).

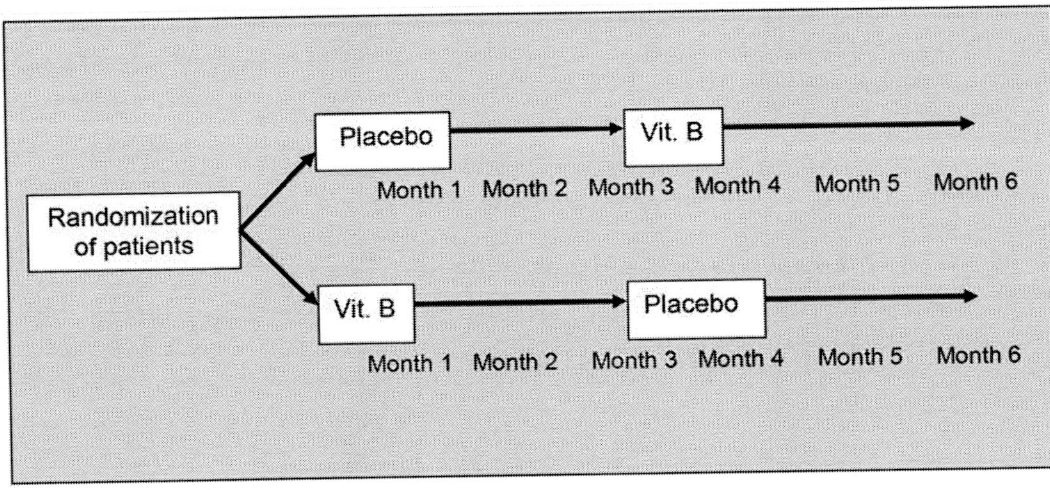

Figure 3. Design of the study titled "homocysteine reducing strategy in schizophrenia".

Forty-two patients completed the study, forty males and two females. This is consistent with previous reports of a much higher incidence of hyper-homocystenemia in male schizophrenics than in female schizophrenics [30, 32]. Twenty-two patients commenced placebo and 20 received active vitamins. All patients entering the study were highly symptomatic but had shown no major clinical changes for at least one month and had no changes in medications in the previous month.

Since this study was not designed to evaluate a new neuroleptic but rather to assess an add-on approach to neuroleptic treatment that was assumed to have a completely different mechanism, changes of up to 20% in the dose of neuroleptics (either an increase or decrease in dose) were allowed at the physician's discretion. While few changes in neuroleptic treatment were made during the period of the study, changes in the administration of neuroleptics (i.m. to oral in an equivalent dose) or in the dose of sedatives, was permitted according to the clinical condition of the patient. The mean length of illness before entering this study was 15.8 years (range 1-39) and mean age was 40 years (range 19-59).

A crossover design was used as an appropriate design for chronic patients in a stable pathologic condition, in an attempt to reduce variance and increase effective sample size. Clinical ratings were done monthly using the Positive and Negative Syndrome Scale (PANSS). Plasma was taken for homocysteine monthly. If patients were discharged, they continued follow-up in a hostel or on an outpatient basis.

Neuropsychological tests were administered by a researcher who was blinded to the patient's condition (placebo/vitamin) at baseline, at the end of three months, and at the end of six months.

Homocysteine levels declined significantly on vitamin therapy compared to placebo in all patients except for one non-compliant subject. Clinical symptoms of schizophrenia as measured by the Positive and Negative Syndrome Scale (PANSS) declined significantly more on active treatment compared with placebo. Of the neuropsychological test, results of the Wisconsin Card Sort (Categories Completed) were significantly better after vitamin treatment than after placebo.

Mean folic acid levels at baseline in these patients were 3.05± .13ng/ml and B_{12} levels were 297±26pg/ml. Correlation of folic acid at baseline with PANSS improvement was -0.27 (p=.08); correlation of baseline B_{12} levels and PANSS improvement was .09 (p= 0.6).

The study thus suggests that a subgroup of schizophrenic patients with hyperhomocysteinemia may benefit from the simple addition of B vitamins.

From our study it is not clear if hyperhomocysteinemia is necessary for the benefits of B vitamin supplementation in chronic schizophrenia. We planned this study assuming that this group be most in need of a reduction in homocysteine levels. However, this should be further tested by a comparison study of B vitamin supplementation in patients with elevated homocysteine vs. patients with normal homocysteine levels.

It is also not clear whether the hyperhomocysteinemia is due to low folate or vitamin B_{12} levels, to polymorphism of methylene tetrahydrofolate reductase (MTHFR), to obesity, or to smoking or excessive caffeine consumption, with any or all of these factors serving as possible markers for the positive benefits of the B vitamins in schizophrenia. We did not measure these variables, this being a limitation of our study.

Since a previous study [33] suggested that environmental factors may explain only part of the variance in homocysteine levels, it is possible that a genetic polymorphism related to homocysteine metabolism may be overrepresented in schizophrenia patients and may be responsible for the interaction with other factors leading to an elevated homocysteine.

CONCLUSION

In general, we suggest that elevated homocysteine may be considered to be a risk factor for schizophrenia, possibly enhancing some of the underlying pathologic processes associated with this condition. The use of homocysteine lowering strategies as an adjuvant to traditional therapy may lead to a further improvement of symptoms, particularly in a subgroup of young male patients exhibiting elevated homocysteine levels.

ACKNOWLEDGMENT

The authors wish to express their gratitude to Prof. Galila Agam for fruitful discussions.

REFERENCES

[1] Selhub J: Homocysteine metabolism. *Annu. Rev. Nutr.* 1999; 19: 217-46.

[2] Grieve A, Butcher SP, Griffiths R: Synaptosomal plasma membrane transport of excitatory sulphur amino acid transmitter candidates: kinetic characterisation and analysis of carrier specificity. *J. Neurosci. Res.* 1992; 32(1): 60-8.

[3] Hoffman DR, Marion DW, Cornatzer WE, Duerre JA: S-Adenosylmethionine and S-adenosylhomocystein metabolism in isolated rat liver. Effects of L-methionine, L-homocystein, and adenosine. *J. Biol. Chem.* 1980; 255(22): 10822-7.

[4] Yi P, Melnyk S, Pogribna M, Pogribny IP, Hine RJ, James SJ: Increase in plasma homocysteine associated with parallel increases in plasma S-adenosylhomocysteine and lymphocyte DNA hypomethylation. *J. Biol. Chem.* 2000; 275(38): 29318-23.

[5] Antun FT, Burnett GB, Cooper AJ, Daly RJ, Smythies JR, Zealley AK: The effects of L-methionine (without MAOI) in schizophrenia. *J. Psychiatr. Res.* 1971; 8(2): 63-71.

[6] Pollin W, Cardon PV, Jr., Kety SS: Effects of amino acid feedings in schizophrenic patients treated with iproniazid. *Science* 1961; 133: 104-5.

[7] Cohen SM, Nichols A, Wyatt R, Pollin W: The administration of methionine to chronic schizophrenic patients: a review of ten studies. *Biol. Psychiatry* 1974; 8(2): 209-25.

[8] Regland B, Johansson BV, Grenfeldt B, Hjelmgren LT, Medhus M: Homocysteinemia is a common feature of schizophrenia. J Neural Transm Gen Sect 1995; 100(2): 165-9.

[9] Regland B, Germgard T, Gottfries CG, Grenfeldt B, Koch-Schmidt AC: Homozygous thermolabile methylenetetrahydrofolate reductase in schizophrenia-like psychosis. *J. Neural Transm.* 1997; 104(8-9): 931-41.

[10] Susser E, Brown AS, Klonowski E, Allen RH, Lindenbaum J: Schizophrenia and impaired homocysteine metabolism: a possible association. *Biol. Psychiatry* 1998; 44(2): 141-3.

[11] Schneede J, Refsum H, Ueland PM: Biological and environmental determinants of plasma homocysteine. *Semin. Thromb Hemost.* 2000; 26(3): 263-79.

[12] Cortese C, Motti C: MTHFR gene polymorphism, homocysteine and cardiovascular disease. *Public Health Nutr.* 2001; 4(2B): 493-7.

[13] Joober R, Benkelfat C, Lal S, et al.: Association between the methylenetetrahydrofolate reductase 677C-->T missense mutation and schizophrenia. *Mol. Psychiatry* 2000; 5(3): 323-6.

[14] Arinami T, Yamada N, Yamakawa-Kobayashi K, Hamaguchi H, Toru M: Methylenetetrahydrofolate reductase variant and schizophrenia/depression. *Am. J. Med. Genet.* 1997; 74(5): 526-8.

[15] Virgos C, Martorell L, Simo JM, et al.: Plasma homocysteine and the methylenetetrahydrofolate reductase C677T gene variant: lack of association with schizophrenia. *Neuroreport* 1999; 10(10): 2035-8.

[16] Wei J, Hemmings GP: Allelic association of the MTHFR gene with schizophrenia. *Mol. Psychiatry* 1999; 4(2): 115-6.

[17] Kunugi H, Fukuda R, Hattori M, et al.: C677T polymorphism in methylenetetrahydrofolate reductase gene and psychoses. *Mol. Psychiatry* 1998; 3(5): 435-7.

[18] Deng H, Liu X, Cai G, et al.: [A linkage disequilibrium study of methylenetetrahydrofolate reductase C677T and schizophrenia]. Zhonghua Yi Xue Yi Chuan Xue Za Zhi 2002; 19(3): 198-200.

[19] Sazci A, Ergul E, Kucukali I, Kara I, Kaya G: Association of the C677T and A1298C polymorphisms of methylenetetrahydrofolate reductase gene with schizophrenia: association is significant in men but not in women. *Prog. Neuropsychopharmacol. Biol. Psychiatry* 2005; 29(7): 1113-23.

[20] Sazci A, Ergul E, Guzelhan Y, Kaya G, Kara I: Methylenetetrahydrofolate reductase gene polymorphisms in patients with schizophrenia. *Brain Res. Mol. Brain Res.* 2003; 117(1): 104-7.

[21] Tan EC, Chong SA, Lim LC, et al.: Genetic analysis of the thermolabile methylenetetrahydrofolate reductase variant in schizophrenia and mood disorders. *Psychiatr. Genet.* 2004; 14(4): 227-31.

[22] Vilella E, Virgos C, Murphy M, et al.: Further evidence that hyperhomocysteinemia and methylenetetrahydrofolate reductase C677T and A1289C polymorphisms are not risk factors for schizophrenia. *Prog. Neuropsychopharmacol. Biol. Psychiatry* 2005; 29(7): 1169-74.

[23] Reif A, Pfuhlmann B, Lesch KP: Homocysteinemia as well as methylenetetrahydrofolate reductase polymorphism are associated with affective psychoses. *Prog. Neuropsychopharmacol. Biol. Psychiatry* 2005; 29(7): 1162-8.

[24] Muntjewerff JW, Blom HJ: Aberrant folate status in schizophrenic patients: what is the evidence? *Prog. Neuropsychopharmacol. Biol. Psychiatry* 2005; 29(7): 1133-9.

[25] Lewis SJ, Zammit S, Gunnell D, Smith GD: A meta-analysis of the MTHFR C677T polymorphism and schizophrenia risk. *Am. J. Med. Genet B Neuropsychiatr. Genet.* 2005; 135(1): 2-4.

[26] Gilbody S, Lewis S, Lightfoot T: Methylenetetrahydrofolate Reductase (MTHFR) Genetic Polymorphisms and Psychiatric Disorders: A HuGE Review. *Am. J. Epidemiol.* 2006.

[27] Lee HC, Jeong YM, Lee SH, et al.: Association study of four polymorphisms in three folate-related enzyme genes with non-obstructive male infertility. *Hum. Reprod.* 2006; 21(12): 3162-70.

[28] Kempisty B, Mostowska A, Gorska I, et al.: Association of 677C>T polymorphism of methylenetetrahydrofolate reductase (MTHFR) gene with bipolar disorder and schizophrenia. *Neurosci. Lett.* 2006; 400(3): 267-71.

[29] Muntjewerff JW, Kahn RS, Blom HJ, den Heijer M: Homocysteine, methylenetetrahydrofolate reductase and risk of schizophrenia: a meta-analysis. *Mol. Psychiatry* 2006; 11(2): 143-9.

[30] Levine J, Stahl Z, Sela BA, Gavendo S, Ruderman V, Belmaker RH: Elevated homocysteine levels in young male patients with schizophrenia. *Am. J. Psychiatry* 2002; 159(10): 1790-2.

[31] Araki A, Sako Y: Determination of free and total homocysteine in human plasma by high-performance liquid chromatography with fluorescence detection. *J. Chromatogr.* 1987; 422: 43-52.

[32] Applebaum J, Shimon H, Sela BA, Belmaker RH, Levine J: Homocysteine levels in newly admitted schizophrenic patients. *J. Psychiatr. Res.* 2004; 38(4): 413-6.

[33] Stahl Z, Belmaker RH, Friger M, Levine J: Nutritional and life style determinants of plasma homocysteine in schizophrenia patients. *Eur. Neuropsychopharmacol.* 2005; 15(3): 291-5.

[34] O'Callaghan P, Meleady R, Fitzgerald T, Graham I: Smoking and plasma homocysteine. *Eur. Heart J.* 2002; 23(20): 1580-6.

[35] Nevo GA, Meged S, Sela BA, Hanoch-Levi A, Hershko R, Weizman A: Homocysteine levels in adolescent schizophrenia patients. *Eur. Neuropsychopharmacol.* 2006; 16(8): 588-91.

[36] Ho PI, Ortiz D, Rogers E, Shea TB: Multiple aspects of homocysteine neurotoxicity: glutamate excitotoxicity, kinase hyperactivation and DNA damage. *J. Neurosci. Res.* 2002; 70(5): 694-702.

[37] Lipton SA, Kim WK, Choi YB, et al.: Neurotoxicity associated with dual actions of homocysteine at the N-methyl-D-aspartate receptor. *Proc. Natl. Acad. Sci. USA* 1997; 94(11): 5923-8.

[38] Moore CS: The real schizophrenia, an abstract life. *Psychiatr. Rehabil. J.* 2001; 25(2): 199-200.

[39] Palmer AM, Marion DW, Botscheller ML, Bowen DM, DeKosky ST: Increased transmitter amino acid concentration in human ventricular CSF after brain trauma. *Neuroreport* 1994; 6(1): 153-6.

[40] Olney JW, Farber NB: Glutamate receptor dysfunction and schizophrenia. *Arch Gen. Psychiatry* 1995; 52(12): 998-1007.

[41] Neeman G, Blanaru M, Bloch B, et al.: Relation of plasma glycine, serine, and homocysteine levels to schizophrenia symptoms and medication type. *Am. J. Psychiatry* 2005; 162(9): 1738-40.

[42] Phillis JW, Smith-Barbour M, O'Regan MH, Perkins LM: Amino acid and purine release in rat brain following temporary middle cerebral artery occlusion. *Neurochem. Res.* 1994; 19(9): 1125-30.

[43] Kruman, II, Culmsee C, Chan SL, et al.: Homocysteine elicits a DNA damage response in neurons that promotes apoptosis and hypersensitivity to excitotoxicity. *J. Neurosci.* 2000; 20(18): 6920-6.

[44] Mattson MP, Shea TB: Folate and homocysteine metabolism in neural plasticity and neurodegenerative disorders. *Trends Neurosci.* 2003; 26(3): 137-46.

[45] Catts VS, Catts SV: Apoptosis and schizophrenia: is the tumour suppressor gene, p53, a candidate susceptibility gene? *Schizophr. Res.* 2000; 41(3): 405-15.

[46] Jarskog LF, Gilmore JH, Selinger ES, Lieberman JA: Cortical bcl-2 protein expression and apoptotic regulation in schizophrenia. *Biol. Psychiatry* 2000; 48(7): 641-50.

[47] Lominadze D, Roberts AM, Tyagi N, Moshal KS, Tyagi SC: Homocysteine causes cerebrovascular leakage in mice. *Am. J. Physiol. Heart Circ. Physiol.* 2006; 290(3): H1206-13.

[48] Kamath AF, Chauhan AK, Kisucka J, et al.: Elevated levels of homocysteine compromise blood-brain barrier integrity in mice. *Blood* 2006; 107(2): 591-3.

[49] Belova I, Jonsson G: Blood-brain barrier permeability and immobilization stress. Acta Physiol Scand 1982; 116(1): 21-9.

[50] Oztas B, Kalkan T, Tuncel H: Influence of 50 Hz frequency sinusoidal magnetic field on the blood-brain barrier permeability of diabetic rats. B*ioelectromagnetics* 2004; 25(5): 400-2.

[51] de Souza FG, Rodrigues MD, Tufik S, Nobrega JN, D'Almeida V: Acute stressor-selective effects on homocysteine metabolism and oxidative stress parameters in female rats. P*harmacol. Biochem. Behav.* 2006.

[52] Dimitrova KR, DeGroot KW, Suyderhoud JP, et al.: 17-beta estradiol preserves endothelial cell viability in an in vitro model of homocysteine-induced oxidative stress. *J. Cardiovasc. Pharmacol.* 2002; 39(3): 347-53.

[53] Huang RF, Hsu YC, Lin HL, Yang FL: Folate depletion and elevated plasma homocysteine promote oxidative stress in rat livers. *J. Nutr.* 2001; 131(1): 33-8.

[54] Yao JK, Reddy RD, van Kammen DP: Oxidative damage and schizophrenia: an overview of the evidence and its therapeutic implications. *CNS Drugs* 2001; 15(4): 287-310.

[55] Dietrich-Muszalska A, Olas B, Rabe-Jablonska J: Oxidative stress in blood platelets from schizophrenic patients. *Platelets* 2005; 16(7): 386-91.

[56] Fendri C, Mechri A, Khiari G, Othman A, Kerkeni A, Gaha L: [Oxidative stress involvement in schizophrenia pathophysiology: a review]. *Encephale* 2006; 32(2 Pt 1): 244-52.

[57] Tosic M, Ott J, Barral S, et al.: Schizophrenia and oxidative stress: glutamate cysteine ligase modifier as a susceptibility gene. *Am. J. Hum. Genet.* 2006; 79(3): 586-92.

[58] Yao JK, Reddy RD, van Kammen DP: Human plasma glutathione peroxidase and symptom severity in schizophrenia. *Biol. Psychiatry* 1999; 45(11): 1512-5.

[59] Nishioka N, Arnold SE: Evidence for oxidative DNA damage in the hippocampus of elderly patients with chronic schizophrenia. *Am. J. Geriatr. Psychiatry* 2004; 12(2): 167-75.

[60] Chen T, Ueda Y, Dodge JE, Wang Z, Li E: Establishment and maintenance of genomic methylation patterns in mouse embryonic stem cells by Dnmt3a and Dnmt3b. *Mol. Cell Biol.* 2003; 23(16): 5594-605.

[61] Rampersaud GC, Kauwell GP, Hutson AD, Cerda JJ, Bailey LB: Genomic DNA methylation decreases in response to moderate folate depletion in elderly women. *Am. J. Clin. Nutr.* 2000; 72(4): 998-1003.

[62] Sato F, Meltzer SJ: CpG island hypermethylation in progression of esophageal and gastric cancer. *Cancer* 2006; 106(3): 483-93.

[63] James SJ, Melnyk S, Pogribna M, Pogribny IP, Caudill MA: Elevation in S-adenosylhomocysteine and DNA hypomethylation: potential epigenetic mechanism for homocysteine-related pathology. *J. Nutr.* 2002; 132(8 Suppl): 2361S-2366S.

[64] Frosst P, Blom HJ, Milos R, et al.: A candidate genetic risk factor for vascular disease: a common mutation in methylenetetrahydrofolate reductase. *Nat. Genet.* 1995; 10(1): 111-3.

[65] Graziano F, Kawakami K, Ruzzo A, et al.: Methylenetetrahydrofolate reductase 677C/T gene polymorphism, gastric cancer susceptibility and genomic DNA hypomethylation in an at-risk Italian population. *Int. J. Cancer* 2006; 118(3): 628-32.

[66] Matsubayashi H, Skinner HG, Iacobuzio-Donahue C, et al.: Pancreaticobiliary cancers with deficient methylenetetrahydrofolate reductase genotypes. *Clin. Gastroenterol. Hepatol.* 2005; 3(8): 752-60.

[67] Egan MF, Goldberg TE, Kolachana BS, et al.: Effect of COMT Val108/158 Met genotype on frontal lobe function and risk for schizophrenia. *Proc. Natl. Acad. Sci. USA* 2001; 98(12): 6917-22.

[68] Bleich S, Junemann A, von Ahsen N, et al.: Homocysteine and risk of open-angle glaucoma. *J. Neural. Transm.* 2002; 109(12): 1499-504.

[69] Sachdev PS, Valenzuela M, Wang XL, Looi JC, Brodaty H: Relationship between plasma homocysteine levels and brain atrophy in healthy elderly individuals. *Neurology* 2002; 58(10): 1539-41.

[70] Bleich S, Kornhuber J: Relationship between plasma homocysteine levels and brain atrophy in healthy elderly individuals. *Neurology* 2003; 60(7): 1220; author reply 1220.

[71] Rao ML, Kolsch H: Effects of estrogen on brain development and neuroprotection--implications for negative symptoms in schizophrenia. *Psychoneuroendocrinology* 2003; 28 Suppl 2: 83-96.

[72] Zandi PP, Carlson MC, Plassman BL, et al.: Hormone replacement therapy and incidence of Alzheimer disease in older women: the Cache County Study. *Jama* 2002; 288(17): 2123-9.

[73] Spence JD, Howard VJ, Chambless LE, et al.: Vitamin Intervention for Stroke Prevention (VISP) trial: rationale and design. *Neuroepidemiology* 2001; 20(1): 16-25.

[74] Godfrey PS, Toone BK, Carney MW, et al.: Enhancement of recovery from psychiatric illness by methylfolate. *Lancet* 1990; 336(8712): 392-5.

[75] Levine J, Stahl Z, Sela B, et al.: Homocysteine reducing strategies improve sympthoms in chronic schizophrenic patients with hyperhomocysteinemia. *Biol. Psych.* 2006; 1(15): 225-227.

In: New Hope for Mental Disturbances
Editors: Vladimir Lerner and Chanoch Meodownik
ISBN 978-1-60692-691-8

Chapter 6

Omega-3 in Psychiatry

Boris Nemets*[1], *Chanoch Miodownik and Vladimir Lerner
Division of Psychiatry, Ministry of Health Be'er Sheva Mental Health Center,
Faculty of Health Sciences Ben-Gurion University of the Negev, Be'er-Sheva, Israel

Abstract

Omega-3 fatty acids are considered essential fatty acids. They are essential to human health, but cannot be manufactured by the body. In recent years, researchers have demonstrated a growing interest in fatty acids and their beneficial influence on human health. Positive findings have multiplied, and more than 500 papers on this topic have been published during the last 70 years. Omega-3 fatty acids are built in to the cell membrane, affecting the function of neurotransmitter receptors. A relationship appears to exist between omega-3 fatty acids and central nervous system (CNS) neurotransmitters. It has been shown that oil diets may have mood-stabilizing effects by reducing the generation of second messengers coming from phosphatidylinositol and phosphatidylcholine in cell membranes. It was suggested that major depression is associated with elevated plasma concentrations of the 2-series prostaglandins (PGE2). Other suggested actions of omega-3 fatty acids include reduction in proinflammatory cytokines, direct inhibition of PKC activity and alteration in serotonergic neurotransmission. Omega-3 fatty acids are believed to stimulate neurotrophic factor, increasing synaptic plasticity, improving neurotransmission, and to have antidepressant and neuroprotective properties.

The History of Omega-3

The history of omega-3 began in the 1700s in Manchester, England. Cod liver oil was used in hospitals in the treatment of patients suffering from arthritis pain. Since the peoples of the Arctic demonstrated little or no health problems within their population, Burr and Burr in

[1] Corresponding author: Boris Nemets, Faculty of Health Sciences, Ben Gurion University of the Negev and Psychiatric Department at Be'er Sheva Mental Health Center. Mail address: Be'er Sheva Mental Health Center, PO Box 4600, Be'er Sheva 84170, Israel. Tel.: +972 8 6401513; Fax: +972 8 6401751;

the 1930s began researching the role of omega-3 in this phenomenon. During the development of modern life, some dietary changes took place, resulting in the absence of omega-3 sources. The trend became widespread all over the world, and negative outcomes (e.g., unwanted health problems) followed [1, 2].

In 1923, the American scientists Burr and Evans discovered that rats deprived of polyunsaturated fatty acids developed symptoms of many illnesses, including hair loss and eczema. They found direct correlation between these problems and deficiency of polyunsaturated fatty acids. In addition to physical problems, some behavioral disturbances are also correlated with fatty acid deficiency. The immune system may become less efficient with resultant slow healing and susceptibility to infections. Evans continued to work with polyunsaturated fatty acids and called them vitamin F, since they were substances vital for bodily function, but ones the body could not manufacture itself.

The fact that alpha-linolenic acid could not correct a deficiency in linoleic acid led Burr a few years later to the conclusion that it was not a single vitamin F, but really two families of essential fatty acids: omega-3, derived from alpha-linolenic acid, and omega-6, derived from linoleic acid [1, 2].

Researchers have shown a growing interest in fatty acids and their beneficial influence on human health. Positive findings have multiplied and more than 500 papers on this topic have been published during the last 70 years.

Omega-3 was originally used by fishermen in the 1970s to rub over their skin to help keep them warm while working in the Icelandic seas. It was well known for its ability to keep the body warm and protect the skin from cracking.

Some researchers have studied Eskimo (Inuit) life. They discovered that coronary heart disease, diabetes, and rheumatoid diseases were present in much lower rates in Eskimos in comparison to their European counterparts. The researchers were surprised to reveal these findings because the Eskimo diet was high in fat from eating animals such as whale, seal, and salmon, which would have have placed them at greater risk from these diseases, rather than less [3-5]. The solution to this conundrum was the discovery that all of the foods that they ate were rich in omega-3 fatty acids, and that this fatty acid is very important for the body in maintaining health.

Molecules

Omega-3 fatty acids are considered essential fatty acids. They are essential to human health but cannot be manufactured by the body. Omega-3 fatty acids are long-chain polyunsaturated fatty acids of plant and marine origin. Fatty acids are divided to three groups according to the occurrence of double bonds in the hydrocarbon chain: saturated fatty acids, which do not have any double bonds in their molecule; monounsaturated fatty acids, which have one carbon-carbon double bond; and polyunsaturated fatty acids (PUFA), which have two or more carbon-carbon double bonds. The omega-3 (ω-3) fatty acids belong to PUFA and are considered essential for normal brain function. Ralph Holman, a researcher studying essential fatty acids, gave omega-3 its name [6].

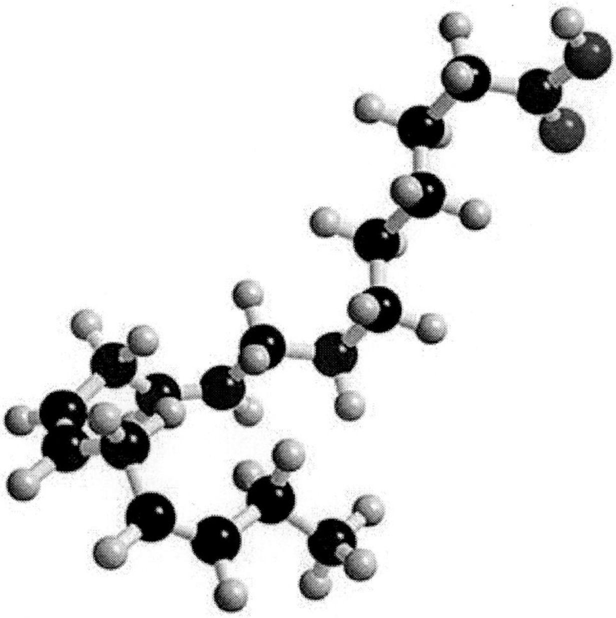

3D model of the omega-3 essential fatty acid structure.

"Omega" is the last letter of the Greek alphabet and initiates a system of notation, which defines the position of double bonds on carbon atoms counted from the methyl (omega) end of the chain. The scheme is based on the detail that double bonds are always separated by three carbon atoms in these molecules. According to the number of carbon atoms, the number of double bonds and the location of the first double bond starting from the omega end of the chain, a fatty acid can be classified. For instance, eicosapentaenoic acid (EPA) is composed of 20 carbon atoms and has five double bonds starting from the methyl (omega) end of the chain (20:5 omega-3). Docosahexaenoic acid (DHA) is composed of 22 carbon atoms and has six double bonds starting from the methyl (omega) end of the chain (22:6 omega-3).

PHYSIOLOGY

Omega-3 fatty acids are built in to the cell membrane, affecting the function of neurotransmitter receptors. A relation appears to exist between omega-3 fatty acids and central nervous system (CNS) neurotransmitters and especially between them and the serotonin system via protein kinase inhibition [7]. It has been shown that, similarly to mood stabilizers such as lithium and valproate which inhibit signal transduction, oil diets may possibly have mood stabilizing effects by reducing the generation of second messengers coming from phosphatidylinositol and phosphatidylcholine in cell membranes [8, 9]. It was suggested that major depression is associated with elevated plasma concentrations of the 2-series prostaglandins (PGE2), which are derived from arachidonic acid (AA) [10]. Omega-3 fatty acids compete with AA, leading to PGE2 reduction and formation of the 3-series of PGs, which are believed to be less inflammatory [11]. Omega-3 fatty acids are included into membrane phospholipids, increasing membrane fluidity, which in turn may reduce the efficiency of phospholipases. In addition, increasing omega-3 fatty acids in membrane phospholipids appears to suppress phosphatidylinositol-associated signal transduction pathways. Other suggested actions of omega-3 fatty acids include reduction in proinflammatory cytokines, direct inhibition of PKC activity and alteration in serotonergic neurotransmission. Omega-3 fatty acids are believed to stimulate neurotrophic factor, increasing synaptic plasticity, improving neurotransmission, and to have antidepressant and neuroprotective properties [12].

Increase of DHA's quantity in brain membrane phospholipids may play a crucial role in membrane fluidity [13]. This theory is supported magnetic resonance imaging [14].

Biological Significances

The possible importance of omega-3 fatty acids was an outcome of observations and studies showing that young humans and experimental animals demonstrated delayed growth when all fatty acids were removed from the diet. Small amounts of omega-3 fatty acids (~1% of total calories) corrected this process and prevented impaired growth [15].

In recent decades, omega-3 has become a subject of interest, since researchers came to the conclusion that there are differences between omega-6 and omega-3 fatty acids. Omega-6 fatty acids (such as γ-linolenic acid and arachidonic acid) play a role in normal growth as well as omega-3; however, they also found that omega-6 was "better" at supporting dermal integrity, renal function, and parturition [16].

There is a competitive effect of omega-3 and omega-6 concerning the activity of its derivates, such as eicosanoids [17]. Eicosanoids made from omega-3 fats often have opposing functions to those made from omega-6 fats (i.e., anti-inflammatory rather than inflammatory). If both omega-3 and omega-6 are present, they will "compete" to be transformed, so the ratio of omega-3:omega-6 directly affects the type of eicosanoids that are produced [18].

This competition was recognized as important when it was found that thromboxane is a factor in the clumping of platelets, which leads to thrombosis [16].

Psychiatric Disorders

Omega-3 fatty acids are known to have membrane-enhancing capabilities in brain cells. It plays a role in the fortification of the myelin sheaths, which is important in neuronal conduction. According to Horrobin, omega-3 fatty acids comprise approximately 8% of the average human brain [19-23]. Holman surmised how omega-3 components are analogous to the human brain by stating that "DHA is structure, EPA is function" [6].

A neuroprotective effect of omega-3 fatty acids helps the brain repair damage by promoting neuronal growth. There are trial descriptions of a structural beneficial impact of omega-3 in some neurological diseases, in comparison to placebo [24].

Some researchers suggest that low brain omega-3 fatty acids in the prefrontal cortex (PFC) of the brain may lower the dopaminergic neurotransmission in this brain area, possibly contributing to the negative and neurocognitive symptoms in schizophrenia. In parallel, reduction in dopamine system function in the PFC may increase dopaminergic function in the limbic system and cause the positive symptoms of schizophrenia. This is the basis for the creation of the omega-3 polyunsaturated fatty acid/dopamine hypothesis of schizophrenia [25]. In pursuing this theory, researchers have tried to examine whether omega-3 supplementation would be effective against both positive, negative and neurocognitive symptoms in schizophrenia. (Further information mentioned below will discuss this issue).

Since omega-3 fatty acid became a focus of research interest in the past two decades, its influence on brain functions became a topic issue as well. Moreover, omega-3 fatty acids were examined in order to reveal their role on mental state and some psychiatric disorders.

Stoll et al. in 1999 published a double-blind placebo-controlled study performed on 30 patients suffering from bipolar affective disorder. Most subjects enrolled in this study were already undergoing psychopharmacological treatment (e.g., 12 out of the 30 patients were treated with lithium). Over the course of four months, the researchers gave 15 subjects capsules containing olive oil, and another 15 subjects capsules containing nine grams of pharmaceutical-quality EPA and DHA. The study showed that subjects in the omega-3 group were less likely to experience a relapse of symptoms in the four months of the study. Moreover, the omega-3 group experienced significantly more recovery than the placebo group [26].

Several epidemiological studies assume that there is an inverse correlation between consumption of seafood and rates of mood disorders. The biological base for this assumption was an indication of deficit in omega-3 fatty acids in people with depressive disorders. Supplementation of omega-3 in several treatment studies demonstrated therapeutic benefits in some of these patients. Deficits in omega-3 fatty acids have been identified as a contributing factor to mood disorders and offer a potential rational treatment approach [27]. Huan and colleagues introduced a study in which they found that EPA levels in red blood cells in suicidal patients were significantly lower than those of the control subjects. According to their results, they suggest that low omega-3 fatty acid levels in tissues are a risk factor of suicide attempt [28]. A similar contribution of omega-3 fatty acids to coronary artery disease may explain the well-described links between coronary artery disease and depression [29-31].

Dietary Sources

Daily Values

The acceptable intake (AI) for omega-3 is 1.6 grams/day for men and 1.1 grams/day for women [32]. The National Institutes of Health recently published recommended daily intakes of fatty acids; specific recommendations include 650 mg of EPA and DHA, 2.22 g/day of alpha-linolenic acid and 4.44 g/day of linoleic acid [33].

Omega-3 supplementation in food has been a significant recent trend in food fortification, with global food companies launching omega-3 fortified bread, mayonnaise, pizza, yogurt, orange juice, children's pasta, milk, eggs, confections and infant formula.

Fish

The most widely available source of EPA and DHA is cold water oily fish, such as salmon, herring, mackerel, anchovies and sardines. Oils from these fish have a profile of around seven times as much omega-3 as omega-6. Other oily fish such as tuna also contain omega-3 in somewhat lesser amounts. Grass-consuming animals have a higher omega-3 profile than grain-fed animals [34].

Not every form of fish oil may be optimally digestible. Of four studies that compare bioavailability of the triglyceride forms of fish oil versus the ester form, two studies did not find a significant difference between them, in contrast to two others that concluded that the natural triglyceride form is better [35, 36].

Although fish is a dietary source of omega-3 fatty acids, fish do not synthesize them; they obtain them from the algae in their diet [37].

Flax

The most available botanical source of omega-3 is flax and its oil. The oil is produced from the plant seeds and which contain omega-3 in amounts six times greater than most fish oils. One tablespoon of ground flax seeds and three tablespoons of water may serve as a replacement for one egg in baking by binding the other ingredients together. Flaxseed oil consists of 55% ALA (alpha-linolenic acid). Flax contains approximately three times as much omega-3 as omega-6 [38]. Fifteen grams of flaxseed oil provides eight grams of ALA, which is converted in the body to EPA and then DHA at an efficiency of 2–15% and 2–5%, respectively [38].

Eggs

Eggs produced by chickens fed a diet of greens and insects produce higher levels of omega-3 fatty acids (mostly ALA) than chickens fed corn or soybeans [33]. Omega-3–enriched eggs provide a dietary alternative to fish for these essential fatty acids. It can provide approximately 1/4 to 1/3 of the recommended intake of omega-3 fatty acids. In addition to feeding chickens insects and greens, fish oils are added to their diet to increase the amount of fatty acid concentrations in eggs [39].

Other Sources

Krill, which are small, shrimp-like zooplankton, also contain the omega-3 fatty acids EPA and DHA, one advantage of extracting omega-3 fatty acids from krill as opposed to sources higher in the food chain [32, 33, 38].

The omega-6 to omega-3 ratio of grass-fed beef is about 2:1, making it a more useful source of omega-3 than grain-fed beef, which usually has a ratio of 4:1 [39]. Milk and cheese from grass-fed cows may also be good sources of omega-3 [32, 33, 38]. One UK study showed that half a pint of milk provides 10% of the recommended daily intake (RDI) of ALA, while a piece of organic cheese the size of a matchbox may provide up to 88% [33, 37].

Microalgae are rich sources of DHA (22:6 omega-3) and can be produced commercially in bioreactors. Oil from brown algae (kelp) is a source of EPA. Walnuts are one of few nuts that contain appreciable amounts of omega-3 fat, with approximately a 1:4 ratio of omega-3 to omega-6 [33, 37]. Acai palm fruit also contains omega-3 fatty acids.

Omega-3 is also found in softgels in pharmacies, and nowadays it is also found in combination with omega-6, omega-9 and shark liver oil [33, 37].

Side Effects

The more common adverse effects of fish oil preparations, particularly in higher dosages, include nausea, fishy belching and looseness of the stools [40]. Because of these effects, the blinding of some of the earlier studies of fish oils in the treatment of mental health problems has been questioned [41]. These problems are much less apparent with purified ethyl ester preparations of omega-3 fatty acids. The safety of omega-3 fatty acids is evident from their acceptance by the regulatory authorities of several countries. For example, the US FDA recognizes the safety of menhaden oil up to a dose of 3 g/day of EPA plus DHA [42], the ethyl esters of EPA plus DHA are registered for prescription in the UK in doses up to 4 g/day [40], and pure ethyl EPA has been marketed in Japan in doses up to 2.7 g/day since 1990.

Most of the other associated effects of omega-3 fatty acids are beneficial, particularly in relation to cardiovascular disease. This is important in a population with mental health problems; patients with both depression and schizophrenia have been shown to be at substantially increased risk of coronary artery disease [43, 44]. Furthermore, some of the commonly used antipsychotic medications, such as clozapine and olanzapine, are associated with elevated plasma triglyceride levels, which are normalized during treatment with omega-3 fatty acids [45].

Omega-3 fatty acids generally do not appear to have clinically significant effects on bleeding time [46], but caution has been urged when using these preparations in high dosages, or for patients with pre-existing hemorrhagic disorders or those on anticoagulant treatment. There have been concerns that omega-3 fatty acid treatment might worsen glycemic control in patients with diabetes mellitus, but this has not been substantiated in two meta-analyses [47, 48].

OMEGA-3 AND DEPRESSION

Depression is a great challenge to every clinician. The conventional antidepressive agents have been researched and developed for more than forty years. However, some depressed patients are non-responders and there are still patients with a negative attitude toward chemical antidepressants. Many studies have been undertaken in order to examine the effect of omega-3 as a single treatment or as additive agent to antidepressive therapy. In the psychiatric literature, uncertainty remains concerning the issue of omega-3 efficacy in the treatment of affective disorders. There are many studies that demonstrate a positive effect, while on the other hand there are some reviews and meta analyses that still lend controversy to this topic [49-53].

A large epidemiological multi-national study by Hibbeln found a negative correlation between fish consumption and depression [54]. The Finnish cross-national study by Tanskanen reported that the chance of having major depression was 31% higher among irregular fish consumers than among frequent consumers. Depressive symptoms were significantly related to irregular fish consumption among women but not among men [55].

Clinical Trials

Six published double-blind placebo controlled trials studied omega-3 fatty acids in major depression. Four of them were designed as add-on studies when the omega-3 was added to ongoing medications [45, 51, 53, 56], while two other trials examined omega-3 as a monotherapy [27, 50]. In the earliest double-blind controlled trial, Nemets and colleagues investigated the effect of ethyl-EPA on 20 patients (all but three of them women) with recurrent major depressive disorder as a supplement to their ongoing medications [51]. It was noted that the patients in this study were best described as having "breakthrough" rather than treatment-resistant depression – they had responded successfully to treatment in the past, but were now experiencing significant symptoms despite adequate ongoing treatment.

Participants were randomized to receive placebo or 2 g/day ethyl-EPA along with ongoing antidepressant therapy for four weeks. By week two, a significantly greater reduction in the Hamilton Depression Rating Scale (HDRS) score in the ethyl-EPA group compared with placebo was observed. EPA treatment had a beneficial effect on so-called core depressive symptoms, such as depressed mood, guilt feelings, insomnia and worthlessness. Peet and Horrobin, in a similar study, examined the effect of ethyl-EPA as an add-on treatment in 70 patients (also mostly females), 18–70 years old, with ongoing depression despite adequate treatment with antidepressants (predominantly SSRIs) [45]. They were randomized on a double-blind basis to receive placebo or ethyl-EPA at doses of 1, 2 or 4 g/day for 12 weeks. Outcome measures were HDRS (17-item version), Montgomery-Asberg Depression Rating Scale (MADRS), and the Beck Depression Inventory (BDI). By 12 weeks, participants who had received the 1-g/day ethyl-EPA as a supplement showed statistically significant improvement comparatively to the placebo group on all rating scales. The 2-g/day and 4-g/day groups showed little evidence of efficacy. Although the authors recommend 1 g/day as a sufficient, effective dose of EPA, there is no basis for the minor efficacy of the higher doses.

Later, Su and colleagues [53] enrolled 28 patients with major depressive disorder in the eight-week double-blind placebo-controlled trial. Patients were randomly assigned to receive capsules providing 4.4 g of EPA and 2.2 g of DHA or placebo in addition to their ongoing antidepressants. Patients receiving omega-3 fatty acids showed significant reduction on the 21-item Hamilton Depression Rating Scale score by week four as opposed to those in the placebo group.

A study was undertaken by Silvers and colleagues [56], who investigated the effects of DHA-enriched fish oil in patients who were treated for depression in a community setting. Seventy-seven patients (18–65 years old) with current depressive episode, without psychiatric co-morbidity, were randomly assigned to receive either 8 g of tuna fish oil (providing 0.6 g of EPA, 2.4 g of DHA and 80 mg vitamin E) or olive oil as placebo, in addition to their ongoing antidepressants, for three months. Outcomes were measured with the nine-item short form of Hamilton Depression Rating Scale (HDRS-SF) and BDI. There was no evidence that fish oil augmentation improved mood compared to placebo. This negative finding was observed despite significant increases in EPA and DHA levels of the RBC membrane phospholipids. Both groups demonstrated significant mood improvement after week two, while a prominent placebo effect was observed. In this trial, high total dosage of the fish oil preparation, which contained only small amounts of EPA versus large amounts of DHA, was used.

Negative findings were also reported in another double-blind, placebo-controlled study for treatment of major depression with DHA [50]. Marangell et al. recruited 36 patients (mostly females) who experienced a non-psychotic major depressive episode (according to DSM-IV criteria) and assessed them using the Montgomery-Åsberg Depression Rating Scale at two and at six weeks. They were randomly assigned to receive either 2 g/day of DHA as monotherapy or placebo for six weeks. The study did not show a significant difference between the DHA and placebo groups in the scale scores at six weeks of treatment.

The last trial by Nemets and colleagues studied the efficacy of omega-3 fatty acids in childhood depression [27]. Twenty-eight children (8–12.5 years old) who experienced a first non-psychotic major depressive episode were randomly assigned to receive either 1 g/d of omega-3 fatty acids or 1 g/d of safflower oil placebo as monotherapy. The omega capsules provided 0.38–0.4 g/d of EPA and 0.18–0.20 g/day of DHA (EPA to DHA ratio of 2:1). Outcome measures included clinician-rated scales (Childhood Depression Rating Scale and Clinical Global Impression) and self-rated scale (Childhood Depression Inventory). Twenty children completed at least one month of the study and were included in the data analysis, according to last-carried forward value (10 from the omega group and 10 controls). Highly significant reduction on all outcome measures was observed in the omega group compared with placebo.

Van Strater and Bouvy [57] studied the literature concerning influence of omega-3 on affective disorders with the help of Pubmed during a 10-year period (1966–2006). The conclusion of this review was that some clinical investigations found that treatment with omega-3 fatty acids did have a positive effect, but the number of test subjects was very limited and some investigations even produced negative results. The authors assume that there is insufficient clinical evidence to prove conclusively that treatment with omega-3 fatty acids has a beneficial effect on affective disorders.

Marangell et al., according to their placebo-controlled study [50], showed that DHA does not demonstrate an antidepressant effect either as a mono or as an augmentation therapy. On the other hand, there is substantial evidence that EPA enhances the effect of antidepressants, providing a new therapeutic option for major depression.

Montgomery and Richardson, in the Cochrane Database Systematic Review, published results from one study that showed positive effects of omega-3 as an adjunctive treatment for depressive but not manic symptoms in bipolar disorder. They suggest dealing with these results cautiously, owing to the limited data available. The authors emphasized that there is an acute need for well-designed and executed randomized controlled trials in this field [58].

Lin and Su performed the latest meta-analysis that showed significant antidepressive efficacy of omega-3 PUFAs. According to their review, it is still premature to validate this finding due to publication bias and heterogeneity. The authors recommend performing more large-scale, well-controlled trials in order to find out the favorable target subjects, therapeutic dose of EPA, and the composition of omega-3 PUFAs in treating depression [59].

Omega-3 and Bipolar Affective Disorder

A large epidemiological research study using data from 11 countries and the Cross-National Collaborative Group (10 countries) studied the lifetime prevalence of bipolar disorder in different countries [60]. A negative correlation between seafood consumption and lifetime prevalence of bipolar I disorder, bipolar II disorder, and bipolar spectrum disorder was revealed. The strongest negative correlation was found between lifetime prevalence of bipolar II disorder (with predominantly depressive symptoms) and seafood/fish consumption. While epidemiological research can hardly prove causality, the findings by Noaghiul and

Hibbeln [60] propose that insufficient ω-3 fatty acid dietary intake may increase the possibility of affective disorders.

Clinical Trials

Omega-3 fatty acids have been studied as a mono-therapy and as an adjuvant intervention in bipolar depression. The following mentioned studies demonstrate that there is a small but significantly greater reduction on the HDRS from either dose compared with placebo; however, no significant effect for mania was achieved [26, 49, 61, 62].

A double-blind controlled preliminary trial conducted by Stoll and colleagues demonstrated a significantly high response in bipolar disorder patients treated with ω-3 fatty acids in comparison with a placebo group [26]. Thirty patients diagnosed with bipolar disorders (types I and II) according to DSM-IV criteria received either 6.2 g of EPA and 3.4 g of DHA or placebo (olive oil) daily as an augmentation to ongoing treatment for four months. The primary outcome measure was the duration of time until deterioration required a change in medication regime. Twelve of fourteen patients in the omega group completed the four-month trial, in comparison with only six of 16 of controls. Kaplan-Meier survival analysis of the study cohort showed that the omega-3–treated group had a significantly longer remission than the placebo one. Secondary outcome measures were the results of Clinical Global Impression, Hamilton Depression Rating Scale, the Young Mania Rating Scale, and Global Assessment Scale ratings, before and after treatment. Significant reduction in scores on Clinical Global Impression, Global Assessment Scale and the Hamilton Rating Scale for Depression was observed in the omega group compared with placebo.

No differences were noted when comparing improvement on the Young Mania Rating Scale (YMRS). Moreover, as noted by Su and Huang [63], the three treatment-emergent mood episodes in the omega group (out of 14 subjects) were mania (1), hypomania (1), and mixed state (1), whereas the 10 episodes in the placebo group (out of 16 subjects) were made up of nine worsening depressions plus one unresolved mixed state. This seems to support Horrobin's original hypothesis that omega-3 might be useful against depression, without suggesting that it might also be useful against mania. Though this trial was criticized for its design [64], statistical analyses used [64], and suitability of using olive oil as placebo [65], its results promised the possible use of ω-3 fatty acids as augmentation treatment for bipolar disorders. Duration of the treatment may be important for the effects of ω-3 fatty acids on mood state to be revealed. A recent study in women with bipolar I disorder showed that a four-week treatment with either a high (5.0–5.2 g/day of EPA, 3.0–3.4 g/day of DHA, and 1.7 g/day of other ω-3 fatty acids) or a low dose (1.3 g/day of EPA and 0.7 g/day of DHA) of ω-3 fatty acids as an add-on therapy significantly increased membrane fluidity. Improvement of membrane fluidity was based on reductions in brain water proton transverse relaxation times (T2) as assessed by magnetic resonance imaging. A dose-dependent effect was observed. However, no significant changes in Hamilton depression scale scores or Young Mania rating Scale Scores were detected suggesting that the biological effects of ω-3 fatty acids were not accompanied by effects on mood state, at least within the four-week treatment [14]. Two double-blind, placebo-controlled trials on adults were conducted by the Stanley Foundation Bipolar Network [49, 66, 67]. In both studies, 6 grams of eicosapentaenoic acid were added to ongoing treatment. In the first study, 59 patients with acute bipolar depression were treated with eicosapentaenoic acid or placebo. In the second study, 62 patients with a rapid cycling bipolar depression were treated with eicosapentaenoic acid or placebo. Both studies showed no significant differences between eicosapentaenoic acid and placebo. The limitations of these studies were lack of placebo effect and prominent severity of recruited patients. Anyway, the results emphasize that the efficacy of eicosapentaenoic acid in bipolar disorder is not yet proven [66, 67].

In conclusion, long-term, large-scale studies involving patients in both acute and chronic phases of bipolar disorders will improve the understanding of the potential of ω-3 fatty acids in the treatment of these disorders. Future studies will also enlighten current concerns that ω-3 fatty acids may be beneficial in depression but not mania and that they may even induce mania or hypomania [63, 68].

Another study supported by the Stanley foundation was performed on children in order to test the effectiveness and safety of omega-3 fatty acids in the treatment of pediatric bipolar disorder (BPD). In this open-label trial, 20 outpatient subjects of both sexes from 6 to 17 years old were enrolled. All of them were diagnosed as suffering from BPD according to DSM-IV criteria. The patients were treated over an eight-week period with omega-3 fatty acids, 1290 mg to 4300 mg combined EPA and DHA. The authors' conclusions were that only 35% of these subjects had positive response. Omega-3 fatty acid treatment was associated with a very modest improvement in manic symptoms in children with BPD [69].

Omega-3 in ADHD and Related Disorders

Attention deficit/hyperactivity disorder (ADHD) is the most widespread neurobehavioral disorder presenting for treatment in youth, although prominent symptoms and impairment often persist into adulthood [70].

Serum levels of docosahexaenoic acid (DHA), dihomo-gamma-linolenic acid (DGLA), and arachidonic acid (AA) were found to be significantly lower in the hyperactive children than in controls [71]. Boys are much more commonly affected than girls, and males are hypothesized to have much higher requirements for EFA than females [72]. As well, approximately 40% of children with hyperactivity had a greater occurrence of fatty acid deficiency symptoms comparative to only 9% of children without hyperactivity. Stevens et al. examined behavior, learning and health problems in six to twelve-year-old boys [73]. Boys with lower plasma levels of ω-3 fatty acids demonstrated a significantly higher incidence of problems associated with EFA deficiency (dry skin, increased thirst, frequent urination) in contrast to subjects with higher levels of ω-3 fatty acids. The Conner's Parent Rating Scales (CPRS-L), Conduct, Anxiety, Hyperactivity/Impulsivity and Hyperactivity Index were significantly greater for children with lower plasma ω-3 fatty acids. Boys with lower ω-3 fatty acids exhibited more common and extreme temper tantrums, and problems getting to sleep and getting up in the morning. More learning difficulties were mentioned in children with lower ω-3 fatty acids. These findings of both clinical signs and biochemical fatty acid abnormalities suggest that intake of ω-3 fatty acids might be helpful in the treatment of ADHD [65]. There are a few randomized double-blind placebo controlled studies evaluating the effects of ω-3 (sometimes in combination with ω-6) fatty acids in children with ADHD. Voigt and colleagues [74] conducted a randomized double-blind placebo-controlled trial on

0.35 g/daily of DHA, as augmentation to on-going stimulant medication, in 54 children six to 12 years old with ADHD. Objectively, inattention and impulsivity were assessed by laboratory measures. For subjective evaluation of children's behavior, two parental behavioral rating scales were also used. As estimated, DHA augmentation increased plasma level of DHA. Nevertheless, no differences were observed between the DHA and the placebo group in ADHD symptoms after the four-month treatment period. These results were additionally confirmed by Hirayama et al., who used a slightly higher dose of DHA [75]. Forty drug-free ADHD children were randomly allocated to either a placebo group or a DHA group for two months. The DHA group received a DHA- fortified diet providing approximately 0.5 g DHA and 0.1 g EPA daily. The control group received identical placebo foods containing olive oil. No significant differences were observed between the two groups. There was just a little improvement of visual and auditory memory for placebo comparative to the DHA group. Following recalculation, it was found that the DHA intervention resulted in significantly reduced aggression in comparison with placebo [76]. Richardson and Puri [77] studied 41 children, eight to 12 years old, with comorbidity of dyslexia and ADHD. During a three-month period they received either a combination of both ω-3 and ω-6 PUFA (daily: 186 mg EPA, 480 mg DHA, 96 mg AA, 60 IU vitamin E, 864 mg cis-linolenic acid, 42 mg AA, and 8 mg thyme oil) or placebo (olive oil). PUFA were significantly better than placebo in reducing cognitive and general behavior problems in the children. In a following study by Stevens et al. [78], children with ADHD and comorbid frequent thirst and skin symptoms were randomly allocated to a PUFA treatment group or placebo (olive oil). The PUFA supplement was enriched in ω-3 relative to ω-6 PUFA and provided 480 mg DHA, 80 mg EPA, 40 mg AA, 96 mg γ-linolenic, 24 mg vitamin E. PUFA supplementation resulted in a significant reduction in the ω-6/ω-3 PUFA ratio in plasma and RBC. No significant difference was observed between the two groups.

A randomized, placebo-controlled trial of dietary supplementation with omega-3 and omega-6 fatty acids was conducted with 177 young children with developmental coordination disorder (DCD) [79]. Treatment during a period of three months in parallel groups was followed by a one-way crossover from placebo to PUFA for an additional three months.

The PUFA group showed significant improvements versus placebo in reading, spelling, and behavior over three months of treatment in parallel groups. After the crossover, similar changes were seen in the placebo-active group, whereas children continuing with active treatment maintained or improved their progress. As suggested by authors, PUFA supplementation may be a relatively safe treatment alternative for learning and behavioral problems among children with DCD.

In recent study by Colter et al., differences in omega-3 fatty acids in dietary intake were examined in order to establish whether this could provide an explanation for the omega-3 abnormalities in red blood cells detected in earlier studies in ADHD adolescents [80]. A secondary idea was to establish whether there were relations between concentrations of omega-3 and particular ADHD behaviors as measured by the CPRS-L. Eleven ADHD adolescents diagnosed according to DSM-IV criteria and 12 age-matched normal controls participated in the study. Blood and dietary intake information, in addition to behavioral assessments, were accomplished. Results showed that ADHD children consumed equal quantities of omega-3 and omega-6 fatty acids to controls, but they had significantly lower levels of total omega-3 fatty acids, higher omega-6 fatty acids and a lower ratio of omega-3:omega-6 fatty acids than the control group. Additionally, low levels of omega-3 fatty acids correlated with higher scores on (CPRS-L). This study hints that ADHD adolescents keep on displaying abnormal omega-3 acid levels that are frequently found in younger children and are definitely different from normal controls of similar age. Moreover, these findings are not explained by differences in intake. This proposes the existence of metabolic differences in fatty acid use between ADHD adolescents and the control group. To conclude, the importance of omega-3 supplements according to this data, remain questionable in ADHD children. Randomized double-blind placebo-controlled trials remain few in number, and thus further studies are needed to prove ω-3 fatty acid efficacy as an alternative or adjunct to conventional treatment options for ADHD. The available evidence so far suggests that supplementation of DHA alone is not effective enough.

Omega-3 Fatty Acids and Schizophrenia

Among numerous theories related to the etiology of schizophrenia, there is the membrane phospholipid hypothesis [21, 22]. The basic idea of this hypothesis is that typical neuronal phospholipid metabolism is essential for normal development of brain construction and function. It was suggested that in schizophrenia there are defects in membrane phospholipid metabolism. These defects include enhanced elimination rates of AA, EPA and DHA from membrane phospholipids, together with a reduced rate of integration of these fatty acids (especially DHA and AA) into phospholipids [21]. The enhanced fatty acid elimination rates have been linked to increased activity of the phospholipase A2 group [21]. Increased PLA2 activity results in loss of essential neural membrane phospholipids, which in turn impairs neural membrane fluidity and, as a result, ion homeostasis, and functioning of membrane-associated proteins and cell signaling systems. The elevated PLA2 activity was demonstrated in the plasma of patients with schizophrenia in comparison with psychiatric and healthy controls [81]. It is interesting, that this activity in schizophrenic patients was normalized after three weeks of antipsychotic treatment [81]. There is no clear evidence on the subject of association between consumption of foods rich in ω-3 fatty acids and schizophrenia [60, 82].

Omega -3 Fatty Acids in Tissues of Patients with Schizophrenia

Trials in postmortem brain tissue have shown phospholipid ω-6 PUFA status abnormalities in schizophrenic patients. Horrobin et al. evaluated postmortem brain samples from seven schizophrenic patients and seven controls. Considerable differences were reported in the phospholipid fatty acid composition in the frontal cortex between schizophrenic patients and normal controls [23]. The main deviation was found in the phospholipid component that is the richest in EFA.

The ω-6 fatty acids (linoleic, γ-linolenic, DGLA, and AA) were all lower than normal in the schizophrenic group, a deficiency to some level compensated by increased quantities of 22:5 ω-6. Significantly reduced levels of ω-6 PUFA (predominantly AA), but not ω-3, were detected in the caudate regions of schizophrenic patients comparative to a control group [83].

Phosphorus magnetic resonance spectroscopy (MRS) is a non-invasive imaging procedure that is utilized for the evaluation of membrane phospholipid metabolism in vivo. Pettegrew et al. originally used MRS to describe membrane phospholipid abnormalities in schizophrenic patients [84]. Eleven drug-naive, first-episode schizophrenic patients were studied and matched up to 10 healthy controls. Schizophrenic patients had significantly decreased levels of phosphomonoesters (PME) and increased levels of phosphodiesters (PDE) in the dorsal prefrontal cortex. This alteration proposed diminished membrane phospholipid synthesis and increased membrane phospholipid breakdown in the medication-naïve schizophrenia subjects. Stanley et al. studied the left dorsal prefrontal cortex of 19 male medicated schizophrenic patients versus normal male controls [85]. Similar to the findings of Pettegrew et al. [84], they published significantly-reduced PME levels in the schizophrenic patients. PDE levels were diminished in the newly-diagnosed patient subgroup demonstrating abnormal metabolism of membrane phospholipids during the early course of schizophrenia. They proposed that this change would be dependent on impaired neurodevelopment around the time of young adulthood, when schizophrenia usually begins.

Clinical Trials

The preclinical findings of abnormal fatty acid composition in membrane phospholipids of schizophrenic patients led to the question of whether ω-3 fatty acid augmentation could be effective in treatment of the illness.

The efficacy of EPA in schizophrenia has been studied in five double-blind controlled trials. Four of them demonstrated little positive results. In a pilot trial, Peet et al. studied EPA as a monotherapy in schizophrenia [86]. Thirty untreated schizophrenic patients diagnosed according to the DSM-IV criteria were included in the trial. Patients were randomly allocated to be treated in a double-blind fashion with either 2 g/day of EPA or corn oil placebo for three months. For ethical reasons, the introduction of conventional antipsychotic medication was permitted when this was considered clinically unavoidable. By the end of the study, all patients in the placebo group required conventional antipsychotic medication. On the other hand, six out of 14 patients in the EPA group remained without antipsychotics at the end of the study. Generally, EPA-treated patients spent little more than a month on conventional neuroleptics contrary to more than two months for the placebo group. Additionally, patients on EPA had lower PANSS scores. Peet et al. evaluated the clinical benefits of 2 g EPA vs. DHA vs. corn oil placebo as augmentation for three months in symptomatic schizophrenic patients [86]. The EPA-treated group showed significantly lower post-treatment scores on the total PANSS than the placebo group; however, there was a remarkable difference at baseline between groups. Using a cut-off point of 25% improvement on the total PANSS score, EPA showed statistical superiority to both DHA and placebo. There was no improvement in negative symptoms. Both of these studies [86] were pilot and therefore their results are not ultimate. In a following trial, Peet and Horrobin [45] studied ethyl-EPA as augmentation therapy in patients with resistant schizophrenia. One hundred and fifteen schizophrenic patients were allocated 1, 2 or 4 g of ethyl-EPA or placebo additionally to their on-going typical or atypical antipsychotics, or clozapine. All patients were symptomatic at the start of the study. After a three-month treatment phase, patients on clozapine showed a significant treatment effect comparative to placebo by taking ethyl-EPA added to their on-going treatment, with an average improvement of 25% in the PANSS scale score. On the contrary, there was no significant difference between ethyl-EPA and placebo when added to other anti-psychotic treatments. The most effective dose of ethyl-EPA was that of 2 g per day, and the effect decreased at the higher 4 g daily dosage. In a study by Emsley et al. [87], 40 symptomatic schizophrenic patients were on 3 g of ethyl-EPA or placebo daily as augmentation to their on-going medicine. By three months of treatment, the EPA group showed a significant decrease in PANSS and Extrapyramidal Symptom Scale dyskinesia scores.

A double-blind, placebo-controlled trial by Fenton et al. had a negative outcome [88]. They recruited 75 chronic schizophrenic or schizoaffective outpatients who were randomly allocated to be given 3 g/day of ethyl-EPA or placebo for a four-month period additionally to their on-going medication. By the end of the study there was no more benefit of EPA supplementation than that of placebo for any of assessed items. To conclude, Joy et al. in the Cochrane Database Systematic Review postulate that the results remain questionable, and omega-3 use in treatment of schizophrenia still remains experimental [89].

Omega-3 and Borderline Personality Disorder

To the best of my knowledge, there is only one controlled trial by Zanarini and Frankenburg [90] studing the efficacy of EPA in borderline personality disorder. The authors conducted an eight-week, double-blind, placebo-controlled monotherapy trial in which 30 women aged 18–40 years with borderline personality disorder were randomly allocated to 1 g/d of EPA (n=20) or placebo (n=10). Subjects meeting criteria for any bipolar disorder or for major depression were excluded from the study. Outcome measures (Modified Overt Aggression Scale and the Montgomery-Asberg Depression Rating Scale) were run at weekly or biweekly intervals. The groups were not statistically different in demographic characteristics, treatment history, or baseline values of outcome measures. EPA was superior to placebo in diminishing aggression as well as the severity of depressive symptoms. Interestingly, this early-onset effect continued until the end of the study, but by week eight both groups improved equally.

Omega-3 during and after Pregnancy

One preliminary open-label trial followed 16 pregnant women with major depression who were randomized to omega-3 FA: 0.5 g/day (n = 6), 1.4 g/day (n = 3), or 2.8 g/day (n = 7) as monotherapy. Subjects averaged reductions of around 50% on the Edinburgh Postnatal Depression Scale and on the Ham-D [91].

Several studies have looked at the possible use of omega-3 in the prevention or treatment of postpartum depression. In one of them, Llorente et al. used only 200 mg/d of DHA during a period of four months after delivery to try to prevent post-partum depressive symptoms; the DHA group did not differ from the placebo group on any measure of depression at the end of the study [92].

Marangell et al. revealed no benefit in the prevention of postpartum depression in a small open-label pilot study (n=7) using 1730 mg EPA + 1230 mg DHA/d (ratio 1.4:1 EPA:DHA) administered approximately one month before and three months after delivery. All women were euthymic when beginning the study, but had experienced postpartum depression in the past; four of the seven developed significant depression during the study [93].

Obsessive Compulsive Disorder

To the best of my knowledge, there is only one placebo-controlled crossover trial of EPA augmentation in obsessive compulsive disorder (OCD) patients [94]. Eleven patients with current OCD according to DSM-IV, on a stable maximally tolerated dose of SSRI and no further improvement for a period of at least two months, were recruited. Subjects were randomly allocated to begin six weeks of placebo (2 g liquid paraffin per day) followed by six weeks of 2 g of EPA daily or six weeks of EPA treatment followed by placebo. Assessments were performed with the Yale-Brown Obsessive-Compulsive Scale (YBOCS), and the Hamilton Rating Scales for Depression (HAM-D) and Anxiety (HAM-A). No significant effect of EPA supplementation was observed, suggesting that adjunctive treatment with EPA is ineffective against OCD.

References

[1] Burr GO, Burr MM. Nutrition classics from *The Journal of Biological Chemistry* 82:345-67, 1929. A new deficiency disease produced by the rigid exclusion of fat from the diet. *Nutr. Rev.* 1973; 31: 248-9.

[2] Burr GO, Burr MM, Miller E. On the nature and role of the fatty acids essential in nutrition. *J. Biol. Chem.* 1930; 86.

[3] Bjerregaarda P, Young K, Hegelec RA. Low incidence of cardiovascular disease among the Inuit—what is the evidence? *Atherosclerosis* 2003; 166: 351-357.

[4] Marshall R. *Arctic Village*. New York: The Literary Guild, 1933.

[5] Allport S. *The Queen of Fats: Why Omega-3s Were Removed from the Western Diet and What We Can Do to Replace Them*. Berkley and Los Angeles: University of California Press, 2006.

[6] Holman RT. The slow discovery of the importance of omega 3 essential fatty acids in human health. *J. Nutr.* 1998; 128: 427S-433S.

[7] Mirnikjoo B, Brown SE, Kim HF, Marangell LB, Sweatt JD, Weeber EJ. Protein kinase inhibition by omega-3 fatty acids. *J. Biol. Chem.* 2001; 276: 10888-96.

[8] Stoll A, Locke C. Omega-3 fatty acids in mood disorders. A review of neurobiologic and clinical actions. In: Mischoulon D,Rosenbaum JF, eds. *Natural Medications for Psychiatric Disorders. Considering the Alternatives*. Lippincott Williams and Wilkins, 2002; 13-34.

[9] Stoll AL, Severus WE. Mood stabilizers: shared mechanisms of action at postsynaptic signal-transduction and kindling processes. *Harv. Rev. Psychiatry* 1996; 4: 77-89.

[10] Calabrese JR, Skwerer RG, Barna B, Gulledge AD, Valenzuela R, Butkus A, Subichin S, Krupp NE. Depression, immunocompetence, and prostaglandins of the E series. *Psychiatry Res.* 1986; 17: 41-7.

[11] Bagga D, Wang L, Farias-Eisner R, Glaspy JA, Reddy ST. Differential effects of prostaglandin derived from omega-6 and omega-3 polyunsaturated fatty acids on COX-2 expression and IL-6 secretion. *Proc. Natl. Acad. Sci. USA* 2003; 100: 1751-6.

[12] Ikemoto A, Nitta A, Furukawa S, Ohishi M, Nakamura A, Fujii Y, Okuyama H. Dietary n-3 fatty acid deficiency decreases nerve growth factor content in rat hippocampus. *Neurosci. Lett.* 2000; 285: 99-102.

[13] Yehuda S, Rabinovitz S, Carasso RL, Mostofsky DI. Fatty acids and brain peptides. *Peptides* 1998; 19: 407-19.

[14] Hirashima F, Parow AM, Stoll AL, Demopulos CM, Damico KE, Rohan ML, Eskesen JG, Zuo CS, Cohen BM, Renshaw PF. Omega-3 fatty acid treatment and T(2) whole brain relaxation times in bipolar disorder. *Am. J. Psychiatry* 2004; 161: 1922-4.

[15] Lands WE. Biochemistry and physiology of n-3 fatty acids. Faseb J 1992; 6: 2530-6.

[16] Das UN. Can essential fatty acids reduce the burden of disease(s)? *Lipids Health Dis.* 2008; 7: 9.

[17] Morrow JD, Hill KE, Burk RF, Nammour TM, Badr KF, Roberts LJ, 2nd. A series of prostaglandin F2-like compounds are produced in vivo in humans by a non-cyclooxygenase, free radical-catalyzed mechanism. *Proc. Natl. Acad. Sci. USA* 1990; 87: 9383-7.

[18] Dreesen TD, Adamson AW, Tekle M, Tang C, Cho HP, Clarke SD, Gettys TW. A newly discovered member of the fatty acid desaturase gene family: a non-coding, antisense RNA gene to delta5-desaturase. *Prostaglandins Leukot Essent Fatty Acids* 2006; 75: 97-106.

[19] Horrobin DF. Essential fatty acid metabolism in diseases of connective tissue with special reference to scleroderma and to Sjogren's syndrome. *Med. Hypotheses* 1984; 14: 233-47.

[20] Horrobin DF. Fatty acid metabolism in health and disease: the role of delta-6-desaturase. *Am. J. Clin. Nutr* 1993; 57: 732S-736S; discussion 736S-737S.

[21] Horrobin DF. The membrane phospholipid hypothesis as a biochemical basis for the neurodevelopmental concept of schizophrenia. *Schizophr. Res.* 1998; 30: 193-208.

[22] Horrobin DF, Glen AI, Vaddadi K. The membrane hypothesis of schizophrenia. *Schizophr. Res.* 1994; 13: 195-207.

[23] Horrobin DF, Manku MS, Hillman H, Iain A, Glen M. Fatty acid levels in the brains of schizophrenics and normal controls. *Biol. Psychiatry* 1991; 30: 795-805.

[24] Puri BK. High-resolution magnetic resonance imaging sinc-interpolation-based subvoxel registration and semi-automated quantitative lateral ventricular morphology employing threshold computation and binary image creation in the study of fatty acid interventions in schizophrenia, depression, chronic fatigue syndrome and Huntington's disease. *Int. Rev. Psychiatry* 2006; 18: 149-54.

[25] Ohara K. The n-3 polyunsaturated fatty acid/dopamine hypothesis of schizophrenia. *Prog. Neuropsychopharmacol. Biol. Psychiatry* 2007; 31: 469-74.

[26] Stoll AL, Severus WE, Freeman MP, Rueter S, Zboyan HA, Diamond E, Cress KK, Marangell LB. Omega 3 fatty acids in bipolar disorder: a preliminary double-blind, placebo-controlled trial. *Arch Gen. Psychiatry* 1999; 56: 407-12.

[27] Nemets H, Nemets B, Apter A, Bracha Z, Belmaker RH. Omega-3 treatment of childhood depression: a controlled, double-blind pilot study. *Am. J. Psychiatry* 2006; 163: 1098-100.

[28] Huan M, Hamazaki K, Sun Y, Itomura M, Liu H, Kang W, Watanabe S, Terasawa K, Hamazaki T. Suicide attempt and n-3 fatty acid levels in red blood cells: a case control study in China. *Biol. Psychiatry* 2004; 56: 490-6.

[29] von Schacky C, Harris WS. Cardiovascular benefits of omega-3 fatty acids. *Cardiovasc. Res.* 2007; 73: 310-5.

[30] Severus WE. Effects of omega-3 polyunsaturated fatty acids on depression. *Herz* 2006; 31 Suppl 3: 69-74.

[31] Parker G, Gibson NA, Brotchie H, Heruc G, Rees AM, Hadzi-Pavlovic D. Omega-3 fatty acids and mood disorders. *Am. J. Psychiatry* 2006; 163: 969-78.

[32] Food and Nutrition Board IoMotNA. *Dietary Reference Intakes for Energy, Carbohydrate, Fiber, Fat, Fatty Acids, Cholesterol, Protein, and Amino Acids.* Washington, DC: The National Academies Press, 2005.

[33] Natoli S. *Literature Review of the Nutritional and Health Benefits of Eggs*. Sidney: Food and Nutritional Australia Pty Ltd, 2005.

[34] ConsumerLab.com PR: Omega-3 Fatty Acids (EPA and DHA) from Fish/Marine Oils. 2005.

[35] Beckermann B, Beneke M, Seitz I. [Comparative bioavailability of eicosapentaenoic acid and docasahexaenoic acid from triglycerides, free fatty acids and ethyl esters in volunteers]. *Arzneimittelforschung* 1990; 40: 700-4.

[36] Lawson LD, Hughes BG. Absorption of eicosapentaenoic acid and docosahexaenoic acid from fish oil triacylglycerols or fish oil ethyl esters co-ingested with a high-fat meal. *Biochemical and Biophysical Research Communications* 1988; 156 960-963.

[37] Whelan J, Rust C. Innovative dietary sources of n-3 fatty acids. *Annu. Rev. Nutr.* 2006; 26: 75-103.

[38] Bartram T. Bartram's Encyclopedia of Herbal Medicine:The Definitive Guide to the Herbal Treatments of Diseases. Robinson Publishing, 1998; 271

[39] Trebunová A, Vasko L, Svedová M, Kasteľ R, Tucková M, Mach P. The influence of omega-3 polyunsaturated fatty acids feeding on composition of fatty acids in fatty tissues and eggs of laying hens. *Deutsche Tierärztliche Wochenschrift* 2007; 114: 275-279.

[40] Mehta D: British National Formulary London: Royal Pharmaceutical Society of Great Britain, 2004.

[41] Damico KE, Stoll AL, Marangell LB, Cohen BM. How blind is double-blind? A study of fish oil versus placebo. *Prostaglandins Leukot. Essent. Fatty Acids* 2002; 66: 393-5.

[42] Administration UFaD: Substances affirmed as generally recognized as safe: Menhaden oil. vol 62, *Fed. Regist.* 1997; 30751-30757.

[43] Brown S, Inskip H, Barraclough B. Causes of the excess mortality of schizophrenia. *Br. J. Psychiatry* 2000; 177: 212-7.

[44] Penninx BW, Beekman AT, Honig A, Deeg DJ, Schoevers RA, van Eijk JT, van Tilburg W. Depression and cardiac mortality: results from a community-based longitudinal study. *Arch Gen. Psychiatry* 2001; 58: 221-7.

[45] Peet M, Horrobin DF. A dose-ranging exploratory study of the effects of ethyl-eicosapentaenoate in patients with persistent schizophrenic symptoms. *J. Psychiatr. Res.* 2002; 36: 7-18.

[46] Eritsland J, Arnesen H, Seljeflot I, Kierulf P. Long-term effects of n-3 polyunsaturated fatty acids on haemostatic variables and bleeding episodes in patients with coronary artery disease. *Blood Coagul. Fibrinolysis* 1995; 6: 17-22.

[47] Farmer A, Montori V, Dinneen S, Clar C. Fish oil in people with type 2 diabetes mellitus. *Cochrane Database Syst. Rev.* 2001: CD003205.

[48] Friedberg CE, Janssen MJ, Heine RJ, Grobbee DE. Fish oil and glycemic control in diabetes. A meta-analysis. *Diabetes Care* 1998; 21: 494-500.

[49] Keck PE, Jr., Mintz J, McElroy SL, Freeman MP, Suppes T, Frye MA, Altshuler LL, Kupka R, Nolen WA, Leverich GS, Denicoff KD, Grunze H, Duan N, Post RM. Double-blind, randomized, placebo-controlled trials of ethyl-eicosapentanoate in the treatment of bipolar depression and rapid cycling bipolar disorder. *Biol. Psychiatry* 2006; 60: 1020-2.

[50] Marangell LB, Martinez JM, Zboyan HA, Kertz B, Kim HF, Puryear LJ. A double-blind, placebo-controlled study of the omega-3 fatty acid docosahexaenoic acid in the treatment of major depression. *Am. J. Psychiatry* 2003; 160: 996-8.

[51] Nemets B, Stahl Z, Belmaker RH. Addition of omega-3 fatty acid to maintenance medication treatment for recurrent unipolar depressive disorder. *Am. J. Psychiatry* 2002; 159: 477-9.

[52] Peet M, Horrobin DF. A dose-ranging study of the effects of ethyl-eicosapentaenoate in patients with ongoing depression despite apparently adequate treatment with standard drugs. *Arch Gen. Psychiatry* 2002; 59: 913-9.

[53] Su KP, Huang SY, Chiu CC, Shen WW. Omega-3 fatty acids in major depressive disorder. A preliminary double-blind, placebo-controlled trial. *Eur. Neuropsychopharmacol.* 2003; 13: 267-71.

[54] Hibbeln JR. Fish consumption and major depression. *Lancet* 1998; 351: 1213.

[55] Tanskanen A, Hibbeln JR, Tuomilehto J, Uutela A, Haukkala A, Viinamaki H, Lehtonen J, Vartiainen E. Fish consumption and depressive symptoms in the general population in Finland. *Psychiatr. Serv.* 2001; 52: 529-31.

[56] Silvers KM, Woolley CC, Hamilton FC, Watts PM, Watson RA. Randomised double-blind placebo-controlled trial of fish oil in the treatment of depression. *Prostaglandins Leukot. Essent. Fatty Acids* 2005; 72: 211-8.

[57] van Strater AC, Bouvy PF. [Omega-3 fatty acids in the treatment of affective disorders: an overview of the literature]. *Tijdschr Psychiatr.* 2007; 49: 85-94.

[58] Montgomery P, Richardson AJ. Omega-3 fatty acids for bipolar disorder. *Cochrane Database Syst. Rev.* 2008: CD005169.

[59] Lin PY, Su KP. A meta-analytic review of double-blind, placebo-controlled trials of antidepressant efficacy of omega-3 fatty acids. *J. Clin. Psychiatry* 2007; 68: 1056-61.

[60] Noaghiul S, Hibbeln JR. Cross-national comparisons of seafood consumption and rates of bipolar disorders. *Am. J. Psychiatry* 2003; 160: 2222-7.

[61] Frangou S, Lewis M, McCrone P. Efficacy of ethyl-eicosapentaenoic acid in bipolar depression: randomised double-blind placebo-controlled study. *Br. J. Psychiatry* 2006; 188: 46-50.

[62] Chiu CC, Huang SY, Chen CC, Su KP. Omega-3 fatty acids are more beneficial in the depressive phase than in the manic phase in patients with bipolar I disorder. *J. Clin. Psychiatry* 2005; 66: 1613-4.

[63] Su KP, Shen WW, Huang SY. Are omega3 fatty acids beneficial in depression but not mania? *Arch Gen. Psychiatry* 2000; 57: 716-7.

[64] Calabrese JR, Rapport DJ, Shelton MD. Fish oils and bipolar disorder: a promising but untested treatment. *Arch Gen. Psychiatry* 1999; 56: 413-4; discussion 415-6.

[65] Puri BK, Richardson AD. The effects of olive oil on omega3 fatty acids and mood disorders. *Arch Gen. Psychiatry* 2000; 57: 715.

[66] Keck PEJ, McElroy SL, Freeman MP, Altshuler LL, Frye MA, Kupka R, Nolen W, Grunze H, Walden J, Denicoff KD, Leverich GS, Post RM: Randomized, placebo-controlled trial of eicosapentanoic acid (EPA) in bipolar depression Fifth International Conference on Bipolar Disorder. Pittsburgh, PA, June 12-14, 2003; *Bipolar Disorders* 2003; 5 [Suppl 1]: P99., 2003; 58.

[67] Keck PEJ, McElroy SL, Freeman MP, Altshuler LL, Frye MA, Kupka R, Nolen W, Grunze H, Walden J, Denicoff KD, Leverich GS, Post RM: Randomized, placebo-controlled trial of eicosapentanoic acid (EPA) in rapid cycling bipolar disorder Fifth International Conference on Bipolar Disorder. Pittsburgh, PA, June 12-14, 2003; *Bipolar Disorders* 2003; 5 [Suppl 1]: P100, 2003.

[68] Kinrys G. Hypomania associated with omega3 fatty acids. *Arch Gen. Psychiatry* 2000; 57: 715-6.

[69] Wozniak J, Biederman J, Mick E, Waxmonsky J, Hantsoo L, Best C, Cluette-Brown JE, Laposata M. Omega-3 fatty acid monotherapy for pediatric bipolar disorder: a prospective open-label trial. *Eur. Neuropsychopharmacol.* 2007; 17: 440-7.

[70] Wilens TE, Biederman J, Spencer TJ. Attention deficit/hyperactivity disorder across the lifespan. *Annu. Rev. Med.* 2002; 53: 113-31.

[71] Mitchell EA, Aman MG, Turbott SH, Manku M. Clinical characteristics and serum essential fatty acid levels in hyperactive children. *Clin. Pediatr.* (Phila) 1987; 26: 406-11.

[72] Colquhoun I, Bunday S. A lack of essential fatty acids as a possible cause of hyperactivity in children. *Med. Hypotheses* 1981; 7: 673-9.

[73] Stevens LJ, Zentall SS, Abate ML, Kuczek T, Burgess JR. Omega-3 fatty acids in boys with behavior, learning, and health problems. *Physiol. Behav.* 1996; 59: 915-20.

[74] Voigt RG, Llorente AM, Jensen CL, Fraley JK, Berretta MC, Heird WC. A randomized, double-blind, placebo-controlled trial of docosahexaenoic acid supplementation in children with attention-deficit/hyperactivity disorder. *J. Pediatr.* 2001; 139: 189-96.

[75] Hirayama S, Hamazaki T, Terasawa K. Effect of docosahexaenoic acid-containing food administration on symptoms of attention-deficit/hyperactivity disorder - a placebo-controlled double-blind study. *Eur. J. Clin. Nutr.* 2004; 58: 467-73.

[76] Hamazaki T, Hirayama S. The effect of docosahexaenoic acid-containing food administration on symptoms of attention-deficit/hyperactivity disorder-a placebo-controlled double-blind study. *Eur. J. Clin. Nutr.* 2004; 58: 838.

[77] Richardson AJ, Puri BK. A randomized double-blind, placebo-controlled study of the effects of supplementation with highly unsaturated fatty acids on ADHD-related

symptoms in children with specific learning difficulties. *Prog. Neuropsychopharmacol. Biol. Psychiatry* 2002; 26: 233-9.

[78] Stevens L, Zhang W, Peck L, Kuczek T, Grevstad N, Mahon A, Zentall SS, Arnold LE, Burgess JR. EFA supplementation in children with inattention, hyperactivity, and other disruptive behaviors. *Lipids* 2003; 38: 1007-21.

[79] Richardson AJ, Montgomery P. The Oxford-Durham study: a randomized, controlled trial of dietary supplementation with fatty acids in children with developmental coordination disorder. *Pediatrics* 2005; 115: 1360-6.

[80] Colter AL, Cutler C, Meckling KA. Fatty acid status and behavioural symptoms of attention deficit hyperactivity disorder in adolescents: a case-control study. *Nutr. J.* 2008; 7: 8.

[81] Gattaz WF, Kollisch M, Thuren T, Virtanen JA, Kinnunen PK. Increased plasma phospholipase-A2 activity in schizophrenic patients: reduction after neuroleptic therapy. *Biol. Psychiatry* 1987; 22: 421-6.

[82] Christensen O, Christensen E. Fat consumption and schizophrenia. *Acta Psychiatr. Scand.* 1988; 78: 587-91.

[83] Yao JK, Leonard S, Reddy RD. Membrane phospholipid abnormalities in postmortem brains from schizophrenic patients. *Schizophr. Res.* 2000; 42: 7-17.

[84] Pettegrew JW, Keshavan MS, Panchalingam K, Strychor S, Kaplan DB, Tretta MG, Allen M. Alterations in brain high-energy phosphate and membrane phospholipid metabolism in first-episode, drug-naive schizophrenics. A pilot study of the dorsal prefrontal cortex by in vivo phosphorus 31 nuclear magnetic resonance spectroscopy. *Arch Gen. Psychiatry* 1991; 48: 563-8.

[85] Stanley JA, Williamson PC, Drost DJ, Carr TJ, Rylett RJ, Morrison-Stewart S, Thompson RT. Membrane phospholipid metabolism and schizophrenia: an in vivo 31P-MR spectroscopy study. *Schizophr. Res.* 1994; 13: 209-15.

[86] Peet M, Brind J, Ramchand CN, Shah S, Vankar GK. Two double-blind placebo-controlled pilot studies of eicosapentaenoic acid in the treatment of schizophrenia. *Schizophr. Res.* 2001; 49: 243-51.

[87] Emsley R, Myburgh C, Oosthuizen P, van Rensburg SJ. Randomized, placebo-controlled study of ethyl-eicosapentaenoic acid as supplemental treatment in schizophrenia. *Am. J. Psychiatry* 2002; 159: 1596-8.

[88] Fenton WS, Dickerson F, Boronow J, Hibbeln JR, Knable M. A placebo-controlled trial of omega-3 fatty acid (ethyl eicosapentaenoic acid) supplementation for residual symptoms and cognitive impairment in schizophrenia. *Am. J. Psychiatry* 2001; 158: 2071-4.

[89] Joy CB, Mumby-Croft R, Joy LA. Polyunsaturated fatty acid supplementation for schizophrenia. *Cochrane Database Syst. Rev.* 2006; 3: CD001257.

[90] Zanarini MC, Frankenburg FR. omega-3 Fatty acid treatment of women with borderline personality disorder: a double-blind, placebo-controlled pilot study. *Am. J. Psychiatry* 2003; 160: 167-9.

[91] Freeman MP, Hibbeln JR, Wisner KL, Brumbach BH, Watchman M, Gelenberg AJ. Randomized dose-ranging pilot trial of omega-3 fatty acids for postpartum depression. *Acta Psychiatr. Scand.* 2006; 113: 31-5.

[92] Llorente AM, Jensen CL, Voigt RG, Fraley JK, Berretta MC, Heird WC. Effect of maternal docosahexaenoic acid supplementation on postpartum depression and information processing. *Am. J. Obstet Gynecol.* 2003; 188: 1348-53.

[93] Marangell LB, Martinez JM, Zboyan HA, Chong H, Puryear LJ. Omega-3 fatty acids for the prevention of postpartum depression: negative data from a preliminary, open-label pilot study. *Depress Anxiety* 2004; 19: 20-3.

[94] Fux M, Benjamin J, Nemets B. A placebo-controlled cross-over trial of adjunctive EPA in OCD. *J. Psychiatr. Res.* 2004; 38: 323-5.

In: New Hope for Mental Disturbances
Editors: Vladimir Lerner and Chanoch Meodownik
ISBN 978-1-60692-691-8

Chapter 7

NOVEL NEUROPROTECTIVE AGENTS FOR SCHIZOPHRENIA: NEUROSTEROIDS, MEMANTINE, BEXAROTENE AND L-THEANINE

***Michael S. Ritsner*•**

Psychiatry Department, the Rappaport Faculty of Medicine, Technion - Israel Institute of Technology, Haifa, Sha'ar Menashe Mental Health Center, Israel

ABSTRACT

Although antipsychotic drugs are an indispensable component of the management of schizophrenia, clinical response of psychopathological symptoms, cognitive impairment, quality of life and elevated emotional distress remains incomplete in schizophrenia. Consequently the development of more effective treatments is an important research goal. One promising direction is the use of neuroprotective agents. This review will focus on the evidence from clinical and basic science studies supporting a role of several potential neuroprotective compounds, representing a wide range of mechanisms, such as neurosteroids (pregnenolone, dehydroepiandrosterone), memantine, bexarotene and L-theanine. Neuroprotective effects of these agents as add-on therapies merit further investigation in schizophrenia and related disorders.

Keywords: schizophrenia, neuroprotective agents, neurosteroids, memantine, bexarotene, theanine

---

• Corresponding author: Michael S. Ritsner, Psychiatry Department, the Rappaport Faculty of Medicine, Technion - Israel Institute of Technology, Haifa; Head, Cognitive and Psychobiology Research Laboratory and Psychiatric Department at Sha'ar Menashe Mental Health Center. Mail address: Sha'ar Menashe Mental Health Center, Israel, Tel: +972 4 6278750; Fax: +972 4 627 8045; Email: ritsner@shaar-menashe.org.il or mritsner@gmail.com.

Abbreviations

AMPA - alpha-amino-3-hydroxy-5-methyl-4-isoxazolepropionic acid
CNS - central nervous system
DHEA - dehydroepiandrosterone
DHEAS - dehydroepiandrosterone sulfate
DHPG - dihydroxyphenylglycine
EPS - extrapyramidal symptoms
$GABA_A$ - gamma-aminobutyric acid
NMDA - N-methyl-D-aspartate
PREG – pregnenolone
PREGS - pregnenolone sulfate

Introduction

Successful treatment of schizophrenia symptoms has not been shown to robustly translate into improvements in cognitive and quality of life deficits, in employment status or social relationships. Beyond the use of antipsychotic agents, it will be of interest to examine whether agents that demonstrate neuroprotective properties in preclinical studies may prove to have neuroprotective effects in schizophrenia. Theoretically neuroprotective approach related to neurodevelopmental, and neurodegenerative models of schizophrenia. These models based on the following findings: (i) MRI studies have revealed brain structural abnormalities from the onset of schizophrenia and the progress of these structural abnormalities; (ii) histopathological studies have elucidated cytoarchitectural abnormalities in schizophrenic brains without gliosis; (iii) obstetric complications are one of the risk factors for schizophrenia; and (iv) relapse of schizophrenia results in a deteriorating progress of the disorder (Murray, 1994; Shenton et al., 2001; Lewis and Levitt, 2002). These models have varied considerably with respect to specificity and timing of hypothesized genetic and environmental 'hits', but have largely focused on insults to prenatal brain development (Rapoport et al., 2005). Longitudinal and cross-sectional studies documented progressive increases in ventricular size, accelerated loss of brain tissues, progressive delays in treatment response, and neurochemical (magnetic resonance spectroscopy) and neurophysiological (P300) indices, all of which are consistent with ongoing cerebral degeneration in a significant subgroup of schizophrenia patients (Knoll et al., 1998). Berger et al. (2003) suggest that dysfunctional regulation of generation, and death of glial and neuronal progenitor cells relevant for neuronal connectivity, and synaptic plasticity are able to reshape our understanding of neurodevelopmental abnormalities, but also underpin an "incipient neurovulnerability" associated with the onset and early course of clinically overt disorders. To account for these findings, McGlashan and Hoffman (2002) propose a pathophysiological model of reduced synaptic connectivity arising from disturbances of brain development active during perinatal and adolescent periods. Thus, the evidence of neural degeneration in the pathophysiology of schizophrenia suggests that there may be treatment opportunities through neural protection.

Promising candidate for neuroprotection therapy should show imitation of brain protective mechanisms. For instance, mechanisms that could impact on gray matter loss include oxidative stress, based on evidence of altered antioxidant levels, changes in the phospholipase A2 system, and glucocorticoid toxicity (Mahadik et al., 2001); mitochondrial dysfunction, based on evidence of reduced mitochondrial numbers and volume (Middleton et al., 2002); on reduced neurotrophic factor support, in which there is decreased brain-derived neurotrophic factor (Hashimoto et al., 2005), and possibly stemming from reduced glial cells numbers in the prefrontal cortex (Stark et al., 2004).

Apoptosis is a one of the most recent mechanisms implicated in the pathophysiology of schizophrenia. Apoptosis is a normal physiologic process that occurs during embryonic development as well as in the maintenance of tissue homeostasis. While apoptosis has normally been associated with neuronal death, its impact can also be sublethal, potentially accounting for neuronal atrophy and synaptic loss without large-scale cell loss. Several postmortem studies have demonstrated that apoptotic vulnerability may be increased in the brains of patients with chronic schizophrenia, even though active cell death is not occurring (Jarskog et al., 2004).

This chapter will focus on a role of pregnenolone, dehydroepiandrosterone, memantine, bexarotene and theanine in neuroprotection.

PREGNENOLONE

Pregnenolone (PREG) and its metabolites such as pregnenolone sulfate (PREGS), dehydroepiandrosterone (DHEA) and dehydroepiandrosterone sulfate (DHEAS), progesterone, allopregnanolone are neurosteroids.

Neurosteroids

The brain traditionally has been considered to be a target site of peripheral steroid hormones. In contrast to this classical concept, new findings over the past decade have shown that the brain itself also has the capability of forming steroids de novo, the so-called neurosteroids (Baulieu, and Robel, 1990). They are synthesized in the central and peripheral nervous system, particularly but not exclusively in myelinating glial cells, from cholesterol or steroidal precursors imported from peripheral sources (Baulieu, 1997; Tsutsui et al., 2006). By comparing the ability of each cell type in the production of neurosteroids, astrocytes are the major producer of DHEA, and androgens, whereas oligodendrocytes are predominantly the producer of PREG and neurons of estrogens (Zwain, and Yen, 1999). At different places in the brain, neurosteroid concentrations vary according to environmental and behavioral circumstances, such as stress, sex recognition, or aggressiveness. Neurosteroids have been implicated as potential signaling molecules for neocortical organization during neuronal development, suggesting that they have trophic factor-like activity (neurotrophic or neurotropic) or can interact with various neurotransmitter systems to promote neuronal remodeling (Mao and Barger, 1998). They have direct effects on major central nervous system (CNS) receptors, especially the gamma-aminobutyric acid ($GABA_A$), N-methyl-D-aspartate (NMDA) and sigma receptors (Majewska, 1992; Debonnel, 1996; Wen et al., 2001). Recent evidence shows that neurosteroids modulate actions on hippocampal neurogenesis (Mayo et al., 2001). As physiologic consequences, neurosteroids are involved in neuronal plasticity, learning and memory processes, aggression and epilepsy, and they modulate the responses to stress, anxiety and depression.

Modes of Action

Current knowledge concerning PREG metabolism, the enzymes mediating these reactions, and their localization has been summarized in recent publications (Compagnone and Mellon, 2000; Stoffel-Wagner, 2003). Briefly, PREG is derived from cholesterol in which the side chain is cleavaged by cytochrome P450scc (Le Goascogne et al., 1987). A physiological function of neurosteroids in the CNS is strongly suggested that PREGS enhances post-training memory processes when injected in very low doses into limbic system structures (Flood et al., 1995). Studies in animals have suggested that PREG and PREGS have “antidepressant” (Reddy et al., 1998) and “anxiolytic” effects (Melchior and Ritzmann, 1994) as well as very potent effects on memory (Flood et al., 1992). More specifically, certain naturally occurring PREG can enhance $GABA_A$ receptor function in a direct manner, and consequently have anxiolytic, analgesic, anticonvulsant, sedative, hypnotic and anaesthetic properties (Belelli, and Lambert, 2005). PREG has neuroprotective effects against both glutamate and amyloid beta protein neuropathology and glutamate neurotoxicity (Gursoy et al., 2001).

Clinical Studies

Clinical studies demonstrated low levels of PREG in the elderly, including those with dementia (Roberts and Fitten, 1990), and in individuals with major depression (George et al., 1994), while depressed women suffering from anxiety-depressive disorder treated with fluoxetine showed significantly higher values of plasma PREG levels compared to the control group (Bicikova et al., 2000). Reported findings demonstrate that male patients (n=8) with generalized anxiety disorder have significantly lower levels of PREGS than control subjects (Semeniuk et al., 2001). Similarly, PREGS levels were significantly lower in 12 non-medicated male patients with generalized social phobia than in 12 matched healthy male controls (Heydari et al., 2002). Serum concentrations of PREGS were significantly lower in 24 patients with hypothyroidism than in age- and sex-matched 43 healthy controls. By contrast, in 22 patients with hyperthyroidism, serum PREGS concentrations were significantly higher (Tagawa et al., 2000). PREG and/or PREGS levels are low in aged humans, including those with dementia (Roberts and Fitten, 1990), and in individuals with major depression (George et al., 1994) and generalized anxiety disorder (Semeniuk et al., 2001).

To investigate the significance of neurosteroids in schizophrenia, we aimed to compare the levels PREG, and DHEA of medicated schizophrenia patients and healthy controls over two months, and to test relationship of these neurosteroids with symptomatology, emotional distress, and anxiety. We repeatedly determined blood levels of PREG, and DHEA in 15 schizophrenia patients and 12 healthy controls. Observations were at four time points: upon entry into the study, and after 2, 4 and 8 weeks. Controlling for age, serum concentrations of PREG were lower (p=0.035), while the DHEA level and the molar ratio values of DHEA/PREG were higher in schizophrenia patients compared to healthy controls (p=0.019 and p=0.014, respectively). The blood levels of PREG appear to be associated with trait-anxiety scores in the schizophrenia patients, while associations of clinical symptoms with two neurosteroids did not reach a significant level when the confounding effect of emotional distress, and anxiety scores was controlled (Ritsner et al., 2006a). Thus, altered serum PREG levels appear to be associated with anxiety and emotional distress scores, but not with schizophrenia symptoms. PREG and DHEA/PREG ratio may represent a trait-like marker of impaired hormonal response to stress in schizophrenia. Although, the role of PREG and DHEA in non-specific response to distress and anxiety or in the pharmacotherapy of schizophrenia is as yet unclear, this report adds evidence to the assumption that, for example PREG and DHEA concentrations, are not related to specific diagnoses, but to more general psychological states, like anxiety, that can occur in various disorders. A further longitudinal large-scale case-control comparison of PREG and DHEA levels in treated and an untreated, as well as, in washed-out schizophrenia patient is warranted.

Recently Marx et al. (2006) investigated neuroactive steroid levels in post-mortem brain tissue from subjects with schizophrenia, bipolar disorder, nonpsychotic depression, and control subjects to determine if neuroactive steroids are altered in these disorders. They found that PREG is present in human post-mortem brain tissue at considerably higher concentrations than typically observed in serum or plasma. Furthermore, PREG was found in the brain, at concentrations of about 1 order of magnitude larger than those of DHEA, as might be expected from a precursor-to-product relationship. The concentrations of PREG and of its sulfate ester (PREGS) were of the same order of magnitude, and about 10-fold larger than in plasma.

Pregnenolone in the Treatment of Psychiatric Disorders

PREG is available over-the-counter in the United States as a nutritional supplement. The therapeutic use of PREG has been considered in neurodegenerative diseases, peripheral nerve damage, epilepsy and substance dependence (Rupprecht, 1997; Akhondzadeh and Stone, 1998; Gasior et al., 1999). Early open-label and placebo-controlled human trials with PREG demonstrated significant improvements in mood, general well-being, psychomotor performance and learning in healthy subjects tested under stressful conditions (Pincus and Hoagland, 1944, 1945; McGavack et al., 1951). Pregnenolone appears to be safe when the dose is between 10 and 100 mg per day (the average PREG production in the body is estimated to be 14 mg per day). In recently study of voluntaries PREG (30 mg per day) also was well-tolerated (Meieran et al., 2004).

Since no evidence of efficacy of PREG augmentation in schizophrenia, the efficacy of pregnenolone in the amelioration of clinical symptoms, cognitive functioning, and improve patients' quality of life in a randomized double-blind, DHEA- and placebo-controlled trial among schizophrenia patients is currently examined (M. Ritsner, V. Lerner, A. Gibel, *ClinicalTrials.gov Identifier NCT00174889*).

DEHYDROEPIANDROSTERONE

DHEA and DHEAS [together abbreviated DHEA(S)] are the major secretory products of the human adrenal glands and brain, and serve as precursors for both androgenic and estrogenic steroids, and also function as neurosteroids that exert multiple effects in the central nervous system and may lead to altered neurotransmission (Akwa, and Baulieu, 2000; Friess et al., 2000; Binello and Gordon, 2003). DHEA is formed from PREG by the microsomal cytochrome P450c17 enzyme (17a-hydroxylase/17,20-desmolase) in the brain and the adrenals (Baulieu, 1998; Zwain and Yen, 1999). DHEA(S) concentrations in the human brain were found to be much higher than in the peripheral circulation but also exceeded their very low CSF levels, ranging from about 1% to 5% of the corresponding plasma concentrations (Guazzo et al., 1996). DHEA(S) levels decrease markedly with age in humans, and levels in elderly populations are reduced to 20% to 30% of peak levels in young adulthood (Nafziger et al., 1998).

Modes of Action

Recent literature has emphasized the unique role that DHEA(S) play in the developing and adult central nervous system (see e.g. Lapchak, and Araujo, 2001; Racchi et al., 2003). Indeed, DHEA appears to cross the blood–brain-barrier (Goodyer et al., 2001) and is also synthesized in the central nervous system (CNS) (Baulieu and Robel, 1996), where it acts together with DHEAS as a weak allosteric antagonist of $GABA_A$ receptors (Majewska et al., 1990) and an agonist of NMDA and sigma 1 receptors (Bergeron et al., 1996). There is evidence supporting a receptor-dependent basis for the direct physiological effects of DHEA(S). The data supporting an intracellular receptor for DHEA(S) are relatively weak and do not allow us to determine whether DHEA(S) directly, or a metabolite of DHEA(S), acts as a direct receptor ligand (Widstrom and Dillon, 2004).

DHEA(S) exhibit anti-stress properties (Hu et al., 2000; Boudarene, Legros, 2002), in particular, as a mediator of the hypothalamic-pituitary-adrenal (HPA) axis adaptation to stress and other psychiatric symptoms (Rasmusson et al., 2003).

DHEA(S) increase neuronal excitability, enhance neuronal plasticity, exhibit reduction of neurodegeneration (Majewska, 1992, 1995), and have neuroprotective properties (Wolf and Kirschbaum, 1999; Lhullier et al., 2004). Studies have shown that DHEA(S) protect certain neuronal populations against neurotoxic insults inflicted by the excitatory amino acid glutamate (Mao and Barger, 1998). Kimonides et al. (1998) have found that DHEA(S) can prevent or reduce the neurotoxic actions in the hippocampus of the glutamate agonists NMDA both in vitro and in vivo or alpha-amino-3-hydroxy-5-methyl-4-isoxazolepropionic acid (AMPA) and kainic acid in vitro. Pre-treatment with DHEA protected primary hippocampal cultures from embryonic day 18 (E18) embryos against NMDA-induced toxicity. DHEA(S) demonstrated neuroprotective effects NMDA-induced neurotoxicity in primary cultured rat hippocampal neurons (Kurata et al., 2004). In addition, DHEA(S) block the neurotoxic effects of cortisol on hippocampal cells (Kimonides et al 1998), protect neurons against glutamate and amyloid ß-protein toxicity (Cardounel et al., 1999), and glucocorticoid toxicity (Kimonides et al., 1999).

Effects of DHEA may be in part mediated by their conversion to testosterone and by the consecutive conversion of testosterone to estradiol by the enzyme aromatase. This enzyme is induced in reactive astrocytes after different forms of neurodegenerative lesions and the resultant local production of estradiol in the brain has been shown to be neuroprotective. The participation of aromatase in the neuroprotective effect of these neurosteroids has been assessed in the study that suggests that estradiol formation by aromatase mediates neuroprotective effects of pregnenolone and DHEA against excitotoxic-induced neuronal death in the hippocampus (Veiga et al., 2003).

Along with neuroprotective effects, DHEA has been shown to display antioxidant properties. DHEA protects hippocampal cells from oxidative stress-induced damage (Bastianetto et al., 1999). DHEA(S) inhibits apoptosis in human peripheral blood lymphocytes through a mechanism independent of either androgen receptors or estrogen receptors (Takahashi et al., 2004), these neurosteroids protect also sympathoadrenal medulla cells against apoptosis via antiapoptotic Bcl-2 proteins (Charalampopoulos et al., 2004).

Next, supplement of DHEA(S) greatly increase neuronal survival and differentiation and reduces astroglial proliferation rates in mouse brain cells in cultures (Bologa et al., 1987). Treating adult male rats with subcutaneous pellets of DHEA increased the number of newly formed cells in the dentate gyrus of the hippocampus, and also antagonized the suppressive of corticosterone. Another word, DHEA regulates neurogenesis in the hippocampus and modulates the inhibitory effect of increased corticoids on both the formation of new neurons and their survival (Karishma and Herbert, 2002).

The question of whether DHEA(S) are related to cognitive functioning was studied in various species. Since the increasing evidence that DHEA has memory-enhancing effects (Roberts et al., 1987; Flood et al., 1992; Migues et al., 2002), it has been hypothesized that DHEA has neuroprotective effects on cognition (Wolf and Kirschbaum, 1999). The specific interaction of DHEA(S) with the hippocampal glutamatergic neurotransmission provided promising mechanism mediating the modulation of cognitive processes. Systemic injections of DHEAS significantly affected the electrophysiological indices of hippocampal plasticity by enhancing the primed burst but not the long-term potentiation in the hippocampus (Diamond et al., 1996). In addition, it has been suggested that an increased glucocorticoid secretion either in response to stressful stimuli or via exogenous administration impairs the hippocampal dependent declarative memory, whereas amygdala-dependent emotional learning appeared to be enhanced by glucocorticoid stimulation (Roozendaal and McGaugh, 1996). The antiglucocorticoid actions of DHEA are particularly interesting with regard to its putative memory enhancing properties.

DHEA in the Treatment of Medical and Psychiatric Disorders

The first clinical investigations produced evidence for an involvement of neuroactive steroids in conditions such as fatigue during pregnancy, premenstrual syndrome, postpartum depression, epilepsy, dementia, depressive and anxiety disorders (reviewed in Stoffel-Wagner, 2001; Pisu and Serra, 2004). There is evidence that therapeutically DHEA might be useful for improving psychological well-being, and for reducing symptomatology in people with major depression (Wolkowitz et al., 1997, 1999), midlife-onset dysthymia (Bloch et al., 1999), systemic lupus erythematosus (van Vollenhoven, 2002), osteoporosis (Sun et al.,

2002), and in patients with advanced HIV infection (Piketty et al., 2001). In all, the range of daily dosages ranged from 50 mg/day to 500 mg/day for 3 weeks to 4 months, with no serious side effects.

More recently, Schmidt et al. (2005) evaluated the efficacy of 6-weeks monotherapy treatment with DHEA (450 mg/d) and 6 weeks of placebo for midlife-onset depression (n=46) in a double-blind, randomized, placebo controlled, crossover treatment study. Significant improvement was observed during DHEA treatment on the Hamilton Depression Rating Scale (HDRS) and the Center for Epidemiologic Studies Depression Scale ratings compared with both baseline (p=0.01) and placebo treatment (p=0.01). Authors concluded that DHEA might be an effective treatment for midlife-onset major and minor depression.

With respect to schizophrenia, three DHEA augmentation treatment studies have been conducted. The first of them compared patients receiving DHEA (n=15) and placebo (n=12) and indicated the significant efficacy of DHEA augmentation (100 mg/day) after six weeks in the management of negative, depressive, and anxiety symptoms of schizophrenia (Strous et al., 2003). Subjects receiving DHEA demonstrated a significant increase in DHEA(S) plasma levels, that were correlated with improvement in negative symptoms, but not with improvement in depressive and anxiety symptoms. Limitations of the small sample size and lack of cognitive and quality of life assessments are noted.

A second study has investigated the effect of DHEA administration during 7 days on medication-induced extrapyramidal symptoms (EPS) among inpatients with schizophrenia or schizoaffective disorder that were randomized in double-blind fashion to receive either 100 mg DHEA or placebo in addition to a constant dosage of antipsychotic medication (Nachshoni et al., 2005). Parkinsonism showed a favorable effect of DHEA with a significant time effect ($p < 0.0001$), as well as a significant group by time interaction ($p < 0.05$) and with no change noted on akathisia. Change of DHEA blood levels was negatively associated with change of Parkinsonism ($p < 0.05$) as well as with change of total EPS ratings ($p < 0.05$). Authors concluded that DHEA appears to demonstrate a significant effect on EPS, with improvement observed particularly in Parkinsonian symptoms.

While the results of these studies were interesting, sample sizes were small and clinical parameters investigated remain limited, we aimed to investigate the effect of DHEA augmentation on symptomatology, neurocognitive functions, side effects, and quality of life in a new group of schizophrenia patients in a large randomized 12-week double-blind, placebo-controlled, crossover trial (Ritsner et al., 2006b). Fifty-five schizophrenia patients were randomly allocated to 2 treatment groups receiving either DHEA (200 mg/day) or placebo for 6 weeks with the crossover between DHEA and placebo occurring after 6 weeks. They continued to receive their regular antipsychotic medication for the duration of the study. Compared to placebo, DHEA administration was associated with significant improvement in cognitive functions of visual sustained attention, visual and motor skills. DHEA augmentation was associated with elevations of both DHEA and DHEAS serum concentrations. DHEA treatment was well tolerated without any serious adverse effects. The study does not confirm previous observations (Strous et al., 2003; Nachshoni et al., 2005) that short-term DHEA augmentation of antipsychotic medication has value in the management of schizophrenia symptomatology and extrapyramidal side effects. However, a long-term, large-scale study with a broader dose range is warranted to further investigate DHEA's role in the management of schizophrenia.

Memantine

Memantine, a NMDA channel blocker, is a member of the aminoadamantane class of organic molecules (1-amino-3,5-dimethlyadamantane). Memantine officially registered for the treatment of Alzheimer's disease (AD)(Wenk, 2006).

Modes of Action

The "glutamate hypothesis" of schizophrenia has emerged from the finding that phencyclidine (PCP) induces psychotic-like behaviors in rodents, possibly by blocking the NMDA subtype of glutamate receptor, thereby causing increased glutamate release (Chavez-Noriega et al., 2002). Multiple lines of evidence have linked abnormalities in glutamatergic receptor expression, subunit composition, and function in schizophrenia (Meador-Woodruff and Healy, 2000; Goff, and Coyle, 2001). Growing evidence suggests that the dysfunction of glutamatergic neurotransmission and of the NMDA receptor may play an important role in the pathophysiology of schizophrenia, especially of the negative symptoms and neurocognitive impairments, and is a promising target for drug development (Wood, 2005). Similarities between behavioral effects of NMDA receptor antagonists and the clinical symptoms of schizophrenia have focused attention on treatment trials targeting a putative hypoactivity of a subpopulation of NMDA receptors. The NMDA receptor channel-complex (composed of NR2 subunits containing the glutamate recognition site and NR1 subunits containing the glycine recognition site) in the postsynaptic membrane senses glutamate and is gated open, provided there are sufficient ambient levels of a glycine-site ligand (Rogawski and Wenk, 2003). NMDA receptor dysfunction in schizophrenia is associated with altered glycine and homocysteine levels (Neeman et al., 2005).

Evidence for hypoactivity of NMDA receptors in schizophrenia has led to therapeutic trials with agents that indirectly activate the glycine modulatory site on the NMDA receptor. Indeed, agents that indirectly enhance NMDA receptor function via the glycine modulatory site reduce negative symptoms and variably improve cognitive functioning in schizophrenic subjects receiving first-generation antipsychotics (Javitt et al., 1994; Heresco-Levy et al., 1999). Clozapine and several conventional agents have been reported to act as partial agonists at the glycine modulatory site of the NMDA receptor, increasing neuronal depolarization at low concentrations and inhibiting depolarization at high concentrations (Banerjee et al., 1995; Lidsky et al., 1997). Consistent with this interpretation, an increase in extracellular glycine attenuated the potentiation by haloperidol of NMDA-receptor-evoked response (Fletcher and MacDonald, 1993). In contrast, long-term administration of antipsychotics may result in desensitization of the glycine modulatory site of the NMDA receptor, as evidenced by a reduction in strychnine-insensitive glycine binding associated with both clozapine and conventional agents (McCoy and Richfield, 1996). These findings suggest that dysfunction of glutamatergic neurotransmission may play an important role in the pathophysiology of schizophrenia, especially of the negative symptoms and cognitive impairments associated with the disorder, and is a promising target for drug development.

Like other NMDA antagonists, memantine causes behavioral activation associated with enhanced cerebral glucose utilization (Butterfield and Pocernich, 2003). Studies have shown that memantine can reverse the decreased metabolic activity associated with AD, possibly accounting for its beneficial effects on cognition and global functioning (Rogawski and Wenk, 2003; Rogawski, 2004). Like other NMDA receptor antagonists, memantine at high concentrations can inhibit mechanisms of synaptic plasticity that are believed to underlie learning and memory. Memantine also has neuroprotective actions in several in vitro and in vivo models (Wenk et al., 1995). Specifically, memantine, at therapeutically relevant concentrations, can protect against neuronal degeneration induced by beta-amyloid (Miguel-Hidalgo et al., 2002). The way in which blockade of NMDA receptors by memantine leads to improved cognitive and psychomotor performance and produces benefits in activities of daily living is unknown. One hypothesis is that there is abnormally enhanced glutamatergic tone in AD that interferes with information processing in neural circuits (Danysz and Parsons, 2003). This glutamatergic tone is associated with mild continuous overactivation of NMDA receptors, which introduces "noise" into the synaptic network and degrades its functional capacity.

Another very different hypothesis is that the cognitive and performance improvement produced by memantine occurs as a result of the psychomotor stimulant and movement-enhancing effects of the drug. In rodents, many uncompetitive NMDA-receptor antagonists including memantine enhance locomotor activity at moderate doses (Schmidt and Kretschmer, 1997).

Memantine in the Treatment of Alzheimer Disease

There have been three randomized placebo-controlled trials demonstrating that memantine is moderately effective in slowing the progression of AD. In the first study, 166 demented nursing home patients (49% AD; 51% vascular dementia) were randomized to 10 mg of memantine or placebo. At 12 weeks the treated patients had improved clinician's global impression scores independent of the etiology of dementia (Winblad, and Poritis, 1999). In another study, 252 patients with moderate to severe AD were randomized to memantine or placebo. At 28 weeks, patients treated with memantine had better activities of daily living function and disability scores. Clinician's impression scores were also improved in the treatment group, but this difference did not reach statistical significance (Reisberg et al., 2003). In the most recent study, 403 patients with moderate to severe AD who were already taking donepezil (stable dose of 5 or 10 mg) were randomized to an additional therapy with memantine or placebo in a blinded fashion. After 24 weeks of follow-up, the memantine-treated group had better cognitive, functional, and behavioral scores compared with the monotherapy group (Tariot et al., 2004). Sleeper (2005) described an antipsychotic-sparing effect observed when memantine was added to the drug regimen of a patient with severe Alzheimer's disease: a 78-year-old white man was receiving risperidone 2 mg 3 times daily for persistent aggressive and dangerous behavioral disturbances. Memantine was initiated, and the dose was titrated to 10 mg twice daily. The patient's response included improvement in functional status and resolution of problematic behaviors, allowing repeated reduction of the risperidone dose and ultimate discontinuation. Thus, memantine has been demonstrated to be safe and effective in the symptomatic treatment of AD (Orgogozo et al., 2002; Rogawski and Wenk, 2003; Potyk, 2005).

Memantine is well tolerated even in long-term therapy with a side effect profile similar to placebo (Winblad, and Poritis, 1999; Reisberg et al., 2003). Reported side effects do not exceed 2%. Common adverse reactions (1-10% and more frequent than with placebo) for memantine and placebo patients respectively were: hallucinations (2.0 vs. 0.7%), confusion (1.3 vs. 0.3%), dizziness (1.7 vs. 1.0%), headache (1.7 vs. 1.4%) and tiredness (1.0 vs. 0.3%). Thus, the data from since 1982 confirm the safety of use and good tolerability profile of this medication at the recommended dosages (10 to 30 mg/day) (Gallarda, and Loo, 2004).

Memantine in the Treatment of Schizophrenia

Two case reports have demonstrated the effectiveness of memantine in a patient catatonic schizophrenia (Thomas, 2005; Carpenter et al., 2006). To the best of our knowledge no findings from clinical trails regarding the use of memantine in schizophrenia have been reported in the literature. There are three ongoing trials aimed to explore the value of memantine in the management of schizophrenia.

- A double-blind, placebo-controlled evaluation of the safety and efficacy of memantine as adjunctive treatment to atypical antipsychotics in schizophrenia patients with persistent residual symptoms (*ClinicalTrials.gov Identifier: NCT00097942*).
- Memantine for the prevention of negative symptomatology and cognitive impairment in schizophrenia (M. Schaefer et al., *ClinicalTrials.gov Identifier NCT00148590*).
- Memantine for the treatment of negative symptomatology and cognitive impairment in schizophrenia (M. Schaefer et al., *ClinicalTrials.gov Identifier NCT00148616*).

BEXAROTENE (TARGRETIN)

Bexarotene (Targretin; LGD1069; 4-[1-{5,6,7,8-tetrahydro-3,5,5,8,8-pentamethyl-2-naphthalenyl} ethenyl] benzoic acid) is a potent RXR-selective retinoic acid agonist with a reduced toxicity profile compared with other nonselective retinoids. After oral administration of targretin capsules, bexarotene is absorbed with a T_{max} of about two hours. Terminal half-life of bexarotene is about seven hours. Bexarotene is highly bound (>99%) to plasma proteins. Four bexarotene metabolites have been identified in plasma: 6- and 7-hydroxy-bexarotene and 6- and 7-oxo-bexarotene. In vitro studies suggest that cytochrome P450 3A4 is the major cytochrome P450 responsible for formation of the oxidative metabolites and that the oxidative metabolites may be glucuronidated. The renal elimination of bexarotene and its metabolites has been examined in patients with Type 2 diabetes mellitus. Neither bexarotene nor its metabolites were excreted in urine in appreciable amounts. Bexarotene is thought to be eliminated primarily through the hepatobiliary system. The pharmacokinetics of bexarotene was similar in men and women. The complex metabolic cascade of retinoids is regulated by enzymatic proteins such as lipoprotein lipases, alcohol dehydrogenases, aldehyde dehydrogenases, and cytochrome P450 enzymes (Dy, and Adjei, 2002).

Modes of Action

Retinoids play a critical role in normal development and physiology by modulating cell growth, division, reproduction, differentiation, and immune function (Sporn, Roberts, 1984). They are also capable of inhibiting cell growth, inducing differentiation, and triggering apoptosis in a variety of tumor cell lines (Martin et al., 1990; Oridate et al., 1996). These effects are mediated by changes in gene expression through nuclear-binding proteins, which act as transcription factors (Leid et al., 1992). There are two types of retinoid nuclear hormone receptors: retinoic acid receptors (RARs) and retinoid X receptors (RXRs). Both belong to the corticosteroid receptor superfamily and co-exist in most cells. The alpha, beta, and gamma subtypes of the RARs and RXRs have distinct and conserved amino and carboxy terminal domains. Each receptor subtype has a specific pattern of expression during embryonal development and a different distribution in adult tissues (Chambon, 1994).

Retinoid receptor (RAR, RXR) families have been shown to mediate genes associated with both growth and differentiation (Gorgun and Foss, 2002). Bexarotene suppresses the thyrotropin [beta] gene promotor by 50%, leading to decreased thyrotropin synthesis and clinical symptoms of hypothyroidism (cold intolerance, depression, and fatigue). Central hypothyroidism resolves with discontinuation of retinoid therapy (Sherman, 2003). Recently, bexarotene was found to induce neuronal differentiation and apoptosis in a variety of preclinical in vitro and in vivo models including cutaneous T-cell lymphoma cells, and has shown efficacy in two multi-centre, open-label Phase II – III clinical trials for early and advanced stages of cutaneous T-cell lymphoma in patients who have failed or were refractory to standard therapies (Querfeld et al., 2006).

Bexarotene in the Treatment of Neoplastic Disorders

Over the last several years, bexarotene has been used to treat a wide variety of neoplastic diseases. For example, since December 1999, targretin capsules have been approved by the FDA for once-daily oral treatment of all stages of cutaneous T-cell lymphoma (CTCL) at an initial dose of 300 mg/m2/day (Hurst, 2000). In addition, bexarotene has been found to be effective in head and neck cancer (Hong et al 1990), advanced non-small-cell lung cancer (Khuri et al, 2001), and metastatic breast cancer (Esteva et al 2003).

Bexarotene is generally administered in doses ranging from 300 - 600 mg/m^2/day, doses that have been found to be effective in clinical trials of neoplastic illness (Hong et al 1990; Rigas et al., 1997). However, the maximum "well-tolerated dose" of bexarotene has been determined as 400 mg/m^2/day (Rigas et al., 1997; Khuri et al, 2001; Smit et al 2003). In clinical trials targretin capsules have been administered for up to 97 weeks.

Targretin capsules and gel are active and generally well-tolerated agents. Most adverse events have occurred at a higher rate in patients treated at starting doses of greater than 300 mg/m^2/day. The adverse events potentially related to treatment include lipid abnormalities (elevated triglycerides, elevated total and LDL cholesterol and decreased HDL cholesterol), hypothyroidism, headache, asthenia, rash, leukopenia, anemia, nausea, increased risk of infection, peripheral edema, abdominal pain, dry skin, dizziness, hyperesthesia, hypesthesia, and neuropathy (Shalita, 1987; Rigas et al., 1997). Hypothyroidism may develop with high-dose bexarotene, most likely because the retinoid X receptor-selective ligand suppresses thyrotropin secretion (Sherman et al, 1999).

Bexarotene in the Treatment of Schizophrenia

At least two hypotheses suggest a rationale for investigation of the possible effect of bexarotene on psychopathology symptoms, cognitive impairment, and quality of life in schizophrenia patients.

First, *the retinoid dysregulation hypothesis* proposed by Goodman (1995, 1998). The following evidence suggests a role of retinoid in the development of schizophrenia. (i) Retinoids are involved in gene regulation and expression and are particularly active in brain neurodevelopment (Satre et al, 1992; McCaffery et al, 1994; Wagner et al., 2002). (ii) Retinoids can influence the expression of receptors for certain hormones and growth factors, and thus can influence the growth, differentiation, and function of target cells by direct and indirect actions. (iii) Retinoids have been shown to directly effect long-term potentiation, direct gating of electrical synapses, and administration of retinoic acid rescues cognitive defects in mice (Chiang et al., 1998; Misner et al., 2001). (iv) Retinoid transcriptional control of schizophrenia candidate genes, e.g., dopamine and glutamate receptors (Arinami et al, 1997; Samad et al, 1997; Krezel, et al, 1998). (v) Increased frequency of retinoid-related minor physical anomalies in schizophrenic pedigrees (Goodman, 1996). (vi) Retinoid toxicity or deficit may result in a symptom profile resembling a severe expression of schizophrenia illness (e.g. enlarged ventricles, thought disorder etc) (Goodman 1998).

Second, *the growth factors deficiency and synaptic destabilization hypothesis* suggests that a functional deficiency of glial growth factors and of growth factors produced by glial cells such as neurotrophins and glutamate leading to a weakening of the synaptic strength may be implicated as one of the important causes of schizophrenia (Moises et al., 2002). A genetically and epigenetically determined low baseline of glial growth factor signaling and synaptic strength is expected to increase the vulnerability for additional reductions. This should lead to a weakening of the positive feedback loop between the presynaptic neuron and its targets, and below a certain threshold to synaptic destabilization and schizophrenia. Authors predict an antipsychotic effect by reducing the synaptic destabilization via the improvement of astroglial function by stimulation of the synaptic protein synthesis rate via glial growth factors.

In our pilot study the effects of bexarotene on severity of psychopathology, cognitive impairment, and quality of life in schizophrenia patients will be examined in an open label design. In this clinical trial, a novel regimen of low dose bexarotene (75 mg/day) was added for 6 weeks to the standard treatment of 25 schizophrenia patients on stable antipsychotic treatment ("Safety and efficacy of add-on oral bexarotene to antipsychotic treatment in schizophrenia patients: an open label trial". V. Lerner, C. Miodownik, and MS. Ritsner; *ClinicalTrials.gov Identifier NCT00141947*).

L-Theanine

L-Theanine (gamma-glutamylethylamide) is a unique amino acid present almost exclusively in the tea plant (*Camellia sinensis*), where it typically occurs in amounts estimated from 1 to 2% by dry weight (Ekborg-Ott et al., 1997). L-Theanine was discovered as a constituent of green tea in 1949 by Sakato, and in 1964 it was approved as a food additive in Japan. Besides being a major source of transportable nitrogen in the root tips, L-theanine is also a precursor for part of the catechin ring system during catechin biosynthesis (Kito et al., 1968). L-Theanine activates the fifth taste sense in the tongue, known in Japanese as *umami*, which roughly translates as deliciousness or brothiness (Ekborg-Ott et al., 1997). It is a water-soluble solid substance with the molecular formula $C_7H_{14}N_2O_3$ and a molecular weight of 160.19 daltons.

Once ingested, L-theanine takes advantage of its resemblance to glutamine to hitch a ride on one of the body's amino acid transporters, a sodium-dependent system that carries L-theanine across the intestine (Kitaoka et al., 1996). In rats, L-theanine is absorbed through the intestinal tract and is hydrolyzed to glutamic acid and ethylamine in the kidney; the peak plasma concentration was found 30 minutes after oral dosing (Unno et al., 1999). When 200 mg of L-theanine was orally administered to rats, the plasma concentrations of L-theanine and ethylamine reached their highest levels about 0.5 and 2 h after administration, respectively. When theanine becomes catabolized in the liver (Bukowski et al., 1999; Terashima et al., 1999) or kidney (Unno et al., 1999; Tsuge et al., 2003), it decomposes into two components: glutamic acid and ethylamine.

It was found that the absorbed L-theanine is transported into the brain through the blood–brain barrier via the leucine-preferring transport system (Yokogoshi et al., 1998a). After passing through the blood brain barrier, theanine is not converted to glutamate by brain-type glutaminase and instead exists as a parent compound (Terashima et al., 1999; Tsuge et al., 2003). It reverts back to its guise as a glutamate mimic and binds to a number of different types of glutamate receptors on nerve cells, although with considerably less affinity than glutamate itself (Kakuda et al., 2002). Recently, Sadzuka et al. (2006) supported the notion that L-theanine acts on the brain-neuron system.

L-Theanine has become as promising candidate for management of schizophrenia because L-theanine may influence neurotransmitters in the brain such as gamma-aminobutyric acid (GABA), dopamine (DA), and serotonin (Yokogoshi et al., 1998a, 1998b), as well as, ameliorates attention and learning (Juneja et al., 1999), emotional distress (Kobayashi et al., 1998), subjective well-being (Okubo et al., 2003), and sleep quality (Ozeki et al., 2002).

Modes of Action

Animal studies have provided evidence indicating that theanine has multiple effects on various neurochemical systems. For example, L-Theanine was reported to trigger dopamine release in the striatum via an interaction with glutamate receptors (Yokogoshi et al., 1998a). Dopamine (DA) is the brain's master regulator of reward and pleasure, and the release of DA probably contributes to the sense of well being associated with theanine intake (or with drinking green tea). Similarly, L-theanine stimulates norepinephrine release, perhaps through its effect of elevating GABA levels, since GABA was reported to increase norepinephrine release in the brain (Kimura and Murata, 1986). Direct administration of L-theanine into the brain striatum by microinjection induced a significant increase of DA release in a dose-dependent manner.

The effect of L-theanine on the serotonin metabolism is more ambiguous, however. One study indicated that L-theanine had no effect on serotonin levels (Kimura and Murata, 1986), whereas two other studies showed that L-theanine decreased serotonin in the brain (Yokogoshi et al., 1995, 1998b). A fourth study reported that theanine elevated serotonin levels in some regions of the brain (Yokogoshi et al., 1998b). Note that taking 5-hydroxytryptophan (5-HTP), along with theanine, may not be especially useful; L-theanine was reported to inhibit the formation of serotonin from tryptophan (Yokogoshi et al., 1998b) and the same could be true for 5-HTP. The concentrations of norepinephrine, 3,4-dihydroxyphenylacetic acid (DOPAC) and 5-hydroxyindole acetic acid (5HIAA) in the brain regions were unaffected by administering theanine except in the striatum (Yokogoshi et al., 1998a). L-Theanine was also reported to induce an inhibition of glutamate reuptake by inhibition of the glutamate transporter (Sadzuka et al., 2001), and to increase GABA concentrations (Kimura and Murata, 1971).

Animal studies also indicate possible neuroprotective effects of L-theanine in the hippocampus through blockade of multiple glutamate receptor subtypes, NMDA, and AMPA (alpha-amino-3-hydroxy-5-methyl-4-isoxazolepropionic acid) receptors (Kakuda et al., 2000; Lu et al., 2004).

The antioxidant activity of L-theanine has been studied with regard to its effect on the oxidation of LDL cholesterol. *In vitro* testing, using malondialdehyde as a marker of lipid peroxidation, demonstrated inhibition of LDL oxidation with L-theanine, although the effect was weaker than the potent antioxidant effect of green tea polyphenols (Yokozawa and Dong, 1997). L-Theanine attenuated the doxorubicin -induced adverse reactions involved in oxidative damage, due to increased glutamate and the recovery of glutathione levels in normal tissues (Sugiyama, and Sadzuka, 2004).

L-theanine may counteract the stimulatory effect of caffeine. In rats, theanine administered intravenously after caffeine dosing, and at approximately the same dose, blunted the stimulant effect of caffeine, documented on electroencephalographic recordings. When given by itself in a smaller dose (20-40% of the original dose), administering theanine resulted in excitatory effects, suggesting that theanine possesses dual activity, depending on the dose (Kakuda et al., 2000).

The main effects of theanine may be grouped as follows: neuroprotective, mood-enhancing, supporting the immune system, possessing anti-obesity and anti-tumor activity, hypotensive, and reducing liver injury effects resulting from alcohol.

Neuroprotective Effects

The neuroprotective effects of L-theanine are the focus of considerable attention. For instance, L-theanine was found to inhibit ischemic delayed neuronal death in gerbils (Kakuda et al., 2000). Furthermore, L-theanine is effective in protecting nerve cells from injury caused by low levels of oxygen, a condition known as ischemia, which is also characterized by excessive glutamate release (Kakuda et al., 2000). L-Theanine was also reported (Sadzuka et al., 1996) to stimulate the release of nerve growth factor (NGF), a protein needed by cholinergic brain cells for survival.

Egashira et al. (2004) examined the neuroprotective effect of L-theanine on ischemic brain damage in a middle cerebral artery occlusion model in mice. Briefly, L-Theanine was injected i.p. 3 h after the occlusion or immediately before and 3 h after the occlusion. Importantly, L-theanine (1mg/kg) significantly decreased the size of the cerebral infarcts 1 day after the occlusion. In contrast, theanine did not affect the cerebral blood flow, the brain temperature, and physiological variables in this model. These results suggest that L-theanine directly provides neuroprotection against focal cerebral ischemia. Although research on brain ischemia has thus far been conducted only in animals, L-theanine holds promise for protecting human brain cells from stroke and from other diseases of glutamate toxicity such as Alzheimer's and Parkinson's.

L-Theanine bears structural similarity to glutamic acid and hence competes with it in binding to glutamate receptors, offering protection against glutamate neurotoxicity (Kakuda, 2002). Additional results suggest that the mechanism underlying the neuroprotective effect of L-theanine is related not only to the glutamate receptor but also to other mechanisms such as the glutamate transporter, although further studies are needed (Kakuda, 2002). Nagasawa et al. (2004) investigated the molecular mechanism underlying the neuroprotective effect of L-theanine using primary cultured rat cortical neurons, focusing on group I metabotropic glutamate receptors (mGluRs). L-Theanine, and a group I mGluR agonist, dihydroxyphenylglycine (DHPG), inhibited the delayed death of neurons caused by brief exposure to glutamate, and this effect of L-theanine was abolished by group I mGluR antagonists. Although administering glutamate alone decreased the neuronal expression of phospholipase C (PLC)-beta1 and -gamma1, which are linked to group I mGluRs, their expression was equal to the control levels upon co-treatment with L-theanine. Treatment with L-theanine or DHPG alone for 5-7 days resulted in increased expression of PLC-beta1 and -gamma1, and the action of L-theanine was completely abolished by group I mGluR antagonists. These findings indicate that group I mGluRs might be involved in the neuroprotective effect of L-theanine. Taken together, these findings strongly support the notion that the neuroprotection by L-theanine can be observed when it is administered orally *in vivo*.

Mood-enhancing Effects

Theanine may have mood-modulating activity and play a role in reducing emotional distress. This amino acid actually acts antagonistically against the stimulatory effects of caffeine on the nervous system (Kakuda et al., 2000; Kakuda, 2002). Research on human volunteers has demonstrated that theanine induces a sense of relaxation in approximately 30-40 minutes after ingestion via at least two different mechanisms. First, this amino acid directly stimulates the brain alpha wave activity (Mason, 2001), creating a state of deep relaxation and mental alertness similar to what is achieved through meditation. Second, the relaxing effects of theanine partly depend on its ability to interact with the brain's glutamatergic system. For example, L-theanine was reported to induce the release of GABA, the main inhibitory neurotransmitter known for counterbalancing the stimulatory effects of glutamate (Kimura and Murata, 1971). Just as glutamate excites nerve cells into greater activity, GABA calms them down. Unfortunately, it is difficult to utilize GABA because it does not traverse the blood-brain barrier readily. L-Theanine, on the other hand, traverses the blood-brain barrier relatively easily. This makes L-theanine rather than GABA itself the supplement of choice for relieving anxiety and stress.

Whereas historically, L-theanine has been shown to have relaxing properties (Juneja et al., 1999; Lu et al., 2004), it also has a reputation for counteracting the anxious jitters associated with caffeine without interfering with its ability to fight fatigue or sharpen mental focus (Kakuda et al., 1996, 2000), although, the anxiolytic effects of theanine have not been established scientifically in animal or human studies. The pharmacological effects of L-theanine reported in animals suggest that it may have some anxiolytic properties, given that both serotonin and GABA play a fundamental role in the neurobiology of anxiety and are molecular targets in the treatment of various anxiety disorders (Kent et al., 2002; Millan, 2003). Supporting the preclinical pharmacological effects of L-theanine, one electrophysiological study using healthy human subjects reported possible relaxing effects of L-theanine (200 mg), as indicated by increased alpha activity in the occipital and parietal cortex (Ito et al., 1998). Although useful, the latter finding does not provide strong evidence for an anxiolytic effect of L-theanine, since alpha activity is regarded as an indirect and crude measure of anxiety, and behavioral measures of anxiety or relaxation were not evaluated and reported. Recently, Lu et al. (2004) examined the acute effects of L-theanine in comparison with a standard benzodiazepine anxiolytic, alprazolam and a placebo regarding behavioral measures of anxiety in healthy human subjects using the model of anticipatory anxiety (AA). Sixteen healthy volunteers received alprazolam (1mg), L-theanine (200 mg), or a placebo in a double-blind placebo-controlled repeated measures study. The findings suggest that although L-theanine may have some relaxing effects under resting conditions, neither L-theanine not alprazolam show any acute anxiolytic effects under conditions of increased anxiety in the AA model.

Other Effects

L-Theanine can affect priming of the immune system (Bukowski et al., 1999; Kamath et al., 2003). When the effects become catabolized into two components (glutamic acid and ethylamine), the glutamic acid is recycled or used as a cellular fuel, whereas any ethylamine not excreted or catabolized continues to circulate. Moreover, ethylamine also happens to be a member of a family of bacterial products (alkylamines) that are recognized by a specific set of T lymphocytes, the γδ cells (Bukowski et al., 1999). T cells of this class ordinarily constitute only 2-5% of all T cells in circulation, but they expand their population by up to 50 times within days of infection by a wide variety of bacteria, viruses, and parasites (Kamath et al., 2003). They similarly increase their numbers when they are primed with alkylamines — including ethylamine derived from tea — and exposed *in vitro* to heat-killed bacteria and parasites or to virus-infected cells. The activated γδ T cells also produce an abundance of antimicrobial cytokines, including interferon gamma and tumor necrosis factor alpha (Kamath et al., 2003).

It was reported that L-theanine might reduce plasma total cholesterol, cholesterol ester, and very-low-density lipoprotein cholesterol (Cooper et al., 2005). Zheng et al. (2004) have demonstrated the anti-obesity effects of L-theanine in mice. Notably, increased body weight and the weight of intraperitoneal adipose tissues were significantly reduced by diets containing L-theanine, and serum concentrations of triglycerides and non-esterified fatty acids were decreased. These results indicated that L-theanine was responsible for the suppressive effect on increased body weight and fat accumulation.

L-Theanine may play a role in modulating the metabolism of cancer chemotherapeutic agents and in ameliorating their side effects (Sadzuka et al., 2000, 2002). In animal tumor models, L-theanine has been found to increase the antitumor activity of some anthracyline agents (doxorubicin, idarubicin) and to ameliorate some of the side effects of these agents. It appears that L-theanine inhibits the efflux of these agents from tumor cells, increasing the inhibitory concentration of the drugs in the target cells. At the same time, L-theanine decreased oxidative stress that these agents induced on the normal cells, possibly due to its mild antioxidant activity. Moreover, L-Theanine can increase the antitumor activity of chemotherapy, even in drug-resistant tumors (Sadzuka et al., 2002) without increasing side effects.

L-theanine has also been shown to lower blood pressure in spontaneously hypertensive rats, although the effect is small and large doses seem to be required (Yokogoshi et al., 1995, 1998c). The lowered blood pressure effect was dose-dependent, with the highest test dose creating the most significant drop. L-glutamine was used as one of the controls. Although L-glutamine is similar in chemical structure to L-theanine, it did not exhibit an anti-hypertensive effect (Juneja et al., 1999).

Dosage and Administration

L-theanine (called Suntheanine®) is protected by over 40 U.S. and international patents for its various physiological efficacies and L-isomer-specific production processes. Based on the results of the clinical studies, L-theanine is most effective in the range of 50-200 mg, with the effect being felt within 30 minutes and lasting for 8-10 hours. For relaxation, 200 mg L-theanine can be taken 2-3 times daily, and a dosage of 400-800 mg three times daily can be used safely. FDA recommends a maximum dose of 1,200 mg per day, although the reason for this limit is not clear, due to its demonstrated safety. L-theanine can also be poured out of the capsule into water, coffee, tea, juice, etc., since it is quickly and completely dissolved. Moreover, L-theanine's potency is not diminished with heat to at least 120° C (100° C is boiling).

Side Effects and Toxicity

L-Theanine appears to be an exceptionally safe nutrient, since it was impossible to find a lethal oral dose even when mice were fed as much as 2 grams per kilogram of body weight (Ueda et al., 2003), which would translate to 140 grams of L-theanine for a human weighing 70 kg. Incidentally, no neurotoxicity of L-theanine itself has been found either in cultured brain cells (Nozawa et al., 1998) or intact animals (Kakuda et al., 2000), confirming theanine's centuries-old record of safety as a food ingredient. Borzelleca et al. (2006)

evaluated the safety of L-theanine (Suntheanine®) when administered as a dietary admixture to male and female rats at concentrations providing doses of 0, 1500, 3000, or 4000 mg/kgbw/day for 13 weeks. There were no consistent, statistically significant treatment-related adverse effects regarding behavior, morbidity, mortality, body weight, food consumption and efficiency, clinical chemistry, hematology, or urinalysis. In addition, there were no consistent treatment-related adverse effects in gross pathology, organ weights or ratios or histopathology. As previously mentioned, L-theanine should be used with caution by anyone undergoing treatment for depression with a selective serotonin reuptake inhibitor (SSRI), since according to some reports, theanine can reduce brain levels of this neurotransmitter (Yokogoshi et al., 1995, 1998b). Pregnant women and nursing mothers should avoid L-theanine supplements. L-theanine is contraindicated in those who are hypersensitive to any component of an L-theanine-containing product.

Relevance of L-Theanine to Schizophrenia

To the best of our knowledge, no clinical trials regarding the use of L-theanine in schizophrenia have been reported in the literature. In keeping with accumulating evidence demonstrating that L-theanine affects neurotransmitter systems related to neurophysiological and disease mechanisms, we hypothesize that L-theanine may play a significant role in ameliorating the expression of schizophrenia symptoms and emotional distress, cognitive dysfunctions, HRQL impairment, and side effects as follows:

It has been hypothesized that negative symptoms are associated with dysfunctional and/or diminished dopamine activity in the prefrontal lobes (Jann, 2004). Thus, since L-theanine also enhances dopamine activity in the central neural system, it is reasonable to assume that L-theanine will be associated with an improvement in negative symptoms. Since the best-documented and the most substantial evidence clearly indicates that L-theanine induces mood-modulating activity and plays a role in reducing emotional distress and anxiety as well as promotes relaxation without causing drowsiness as described above, it seems worthwhile to investigate the efficacy of L-theanine in the management of mood and emotional distress symptoms in schizophrenia. This becomes particularly relevant considering the high incidence of affective symptomatology in patients with schizophrenia and the high rate of suicidal behavior; approximately 50% attempt suicide and 10% successfully commit suicide.

Although investigation of the use of L-theanine has not provided definitive evidence of its positive effects in improving cognitive dysfunction, preliminary investigation indicates that L-theanine has some potential benefit in improving attention and learning, as well as in heightening mental acuity (Juneja et al., 1999). It has been suggested that individuals with cognitive deficits may benefit from receiving L-theanine. Although the rationale for expecting similar cognitive improvement in schizophrenia individuals remains somewhat weak and untested, the possibility certainly exists. Thus, whether these benefits may be extended to improvement of neurocognitive dysfunction in schizophrenia remains unknown, but it certainly merits at least a preliminary pilot investigation.

Since administering L-theanine has resulted in positive effects on subjective well-being (Okubo et al., 2003) and sleep quality (Ozeki et al., 2002), it appears prudent to consider the potential positive effects of L-theanine in the management of quality of life impairment in schizophrenia. At least two studies have demonstrated anti-obesity effects following L-theanine administration (Zheng et al., 2004; Cooper et al., 2005), which may be useful for ameliorating the metabolic side effects of antipsychotic agent symptoms.

The first study of the effects of L-theanine in male child subjects with attention deficit hyperactivity disorder has been started at October 2005 (M. Lyon, *ClinicalTrials.gov Identifier NCT00291070*). Currently we examine the value of L-theanine in treatment of schizophrenia and schizoaffective disorders. This is a two-year randomized placebo-controlled double-blind investigation of the use of augmentative L-theanine (Suntheanine®) in the management of 60 patients. Participating subjects on stable antipsychotic treatment will be randomized to receive for 8 weeks either L-theanine (Suntheanine®; 400 mg/day) or a placebo in addition to regular ongoing antipsychotic medication for 8 weeks. Subjects will be assessed at baseline and after 2, 4, 6, and 8 weeks of treatment using psychiatric rating scales, self-reported questionnaires, and a neuropsychological battery of tests. Outcome variables include the severity of symptoms, and emotional distress, cognitive functioning, side effects, and the quality of life. The efficacy and safety of augmenting antipsychotic treatment with L-theanine will be analyzed. The results of this research study may identify an agent capable of improving the symptoms, the neurocognitive deficit, distress symptoms, side effects, and the quality of life of patients with schizophrenia.

NEUROPROTECTION

In recent years neuroprotection has been used as a novel approach to the treatment of schizophrenia, since accumulating evidence suggests that the progressive course of the illness is associated with ongoing neurodegenerative processes. Ehrenreich, and Siren (2001) defined neuroprotection as the effort to maintain the highest possible intactness of cellular interactions or intercellular communication in the brain resulting in an overall undisturbed function. In other words, neuroprotection actually means protection of neural function, and refers to treatment that helps to maintain the functional integrity of the CNS in response to neurobiological stress. Therefore, beyond the use of antipsychotic agents, it will be of interest to examine whether agents that demonstrate neuroprotective properties in preclinical studies may prove to have neuroprotective effects in clinical trials. In contrast to conventional interventions, a neuroprotection approach suggests applying neuroprotective agents as "add-on therapy" to the antipsychotic treatment.

With the exception of dementia, the use of neuroprotective agents in psychiatric disorders is not yet well established. Neuroprotective agents as add-on therapies (e.g., modafinil, erythropoietin, glycine, D-serine, memantine and celecoxib) are currently being evaluated in schizophrenia and related disorders (see review: Krebs et al., 2006). One of the oldest and most successful agents used in psychiatry, lithium, can be viewed as a prototype of such a neuroprotective agent (Manji et al., 1999). Ehrenreich et al. (2004) reviewed the neuroprotective approach using erythropoietin (EPO; that is a natural body-own-protein hormone that has been used for treatment of anemia) represents a totally new frontier. The "Gottingen EPO-stroke trial" represents the first effective use in man of a neuroprotective therapy in an acute brain disease while the experimental EPO therapy to combat cognitive decline in patients with schizophrenia will be introduced as an example of a neuroprotective strategy for a chronic brain disease. There is ample evidence that neurotrophins (Lang et al.,

2004) and endogenous cannabinoid system (Gambi et al., 2005) have numerous neuroprotective effects. This chapter highlights recent evidence from clinical and basic science studies supporting a role for pregnenolone, dehydroepiandrosterone, memantine, bexarotene and L-theanine in neuroprotection. The mechanisms underlying neuroprotective effects of these compounds are various and independent of the classically defined dopamine and serotonin receptors. Neuroprotective effects of these agents as add-on therapies merit further investigation in schizophrenia and related disorders.

ACKNOWLEDGMENTS

This work was partly supported by generous grants from the Stanley Foundation (02T-229 and 05T-648). The author would like to express gratitude to Drs. Anatoly Gibel, Yael Ratner, Vladimir Lerner, Rachel Maayan, Rael Strous, Tzvi Dwolatzky, and Abracham Weizman for fruitful cooperation.

REFERENCES

Akhondzadeh, S., Stone, T.W. Potentiation of muscimol-induced long-term depression by benzodiazepines and prevention or reversal by pregnenolone sulfate. *Pharmacol. Res.,* 1998, 38, 441–448.

Akwa Y, Baulieu EE. Dehydroepiandrosterone sulfate and dehydroepiandrosterone: neuroactive neurosteroids. *Current Opinion in Endocrinology and Diabetes*, 2000, 7,160-167.

Arinami T, Gao M, Hamaguchi H, Toru M. A functional polymorphism in the promoter region of the dopamine D2 receptor gene is associated with schizophrenia. *Human Molecular Genetics*, 1997, 6, 577-582.

Banerjee SP, Zuck LG, Yablonsky-Alter E, Lidsky TI. Glutamate agonist activity: implications for antipsychotic drug action and schizophrenia. *Neuroreport*, 1995, 6, 2500-2504.

Bastianetto S, Ramassamy C, Poirier J, Quirion R. Dehydroepiandrosterone (DHEA) protects hippocampal cells from oxidative stress-induced damage. *Brain Res. Mol. Brain Res.*, 1999, 20, 66, 35-41.

Baulieu EE , Robel P. Neurosteroids: a new brain function? *Journal of Steroid Biochemistry and Molecular Biology,* 1990, 37, 395-403.

Baulieu EE, Robel P. Dehydroepiandrosterone and dehydroepiandrosterone sulfate as neuroactive neurosteroids. *Journal of Endocrinology*, 1996, 50, 221–239.

Baulieu, E.E. Neurosteroids: of the nervous system, by the nervous system, for the nervous system. *Recent Prog.. in Hormone Res.*, 1997, 52, 1-32.

Baulieu, E.E. Neurosteroids: a novel function of the brain. *Psychoneuroendocrinology*, 1998, 23, 963–987.

Belelli D, Lambert JJ. Neurosteroids: endogenous regulators of the GABA(A) receptor. *Nat. Rev. Neurosci.*, 2005,,6,,565-75.

Berger GE, Wood S, McGorry PD. Incipient neurovulnerability and neuroprotection in early psychosis. *Psychopharmacol. Bull.*, 2003, 37, 79-101.

Bergeron R, de Montigny C, Debonnel G, Potentiationof neuronal NMDA response induced by dehydroepiandrosterone and its suppression by progesterone: effects mediated via sigma receptors. *Journal of Neuroscience*, 1996, 16, 193–202.

Bicikova, M., Tallova, J., Hill, M., Krausova, Z. and Hampl, R. Serum concentrations of some neuroactive steroids in women suffering from mixed anxiety-depressive disorder. *Neurochem. Res.,* 2000, 25, 1623-1627.

Binello E, Gordon CM. Clinical uses and misuses of dehydroepiandrosterone. *Curr. Opin. Pharmacol.*, 2003, 3, 635-41.

Bloch M, Schmidt PJ, Danaceau MA, Adams LF, Rubinow DR. Dehydroepiandrosterone treatment of midlife dysthymia. *Biol. Psychiatry*,1999, 45, 1533-41.

Bologa L, Sharma J, Roberts E. Dehydroepiandrosterone and its sulfated derivative reduce neuronal death and enhance astrocytic differentiation in brain cell cultures. *J. Neurosci. Res.,* 1987,17, 225-34.

Borzelleca JF, Peters D, Hall W. A 13-week dietary toxicity and toxicokinetic study with l-theanine in rats. *Food Chem. Toxicol.,* 2006, [Epub ahead of print]

Boudarene M, Legros JJ. Boudarene M, Legros JJ, Timsit-Berthier M. Study of the stress response: role of anxiety, cortisol and DHEA-S. *Encephale*, 2002, 28,139-46.

Bukowski JF, Morita CT, Brenner MB. Human γδ T cells recognize alkylamines derived from microbes, edible plants, and tea: implications for innate immunity. *Immunity,* 1999,11, 57-65.

Butterfield DA, Pocernich CB. The glutamatergic system and Alzheimer's disease: therapeutic implications. *CNS Drugs,* 2003,17, 641– 652.

Cardounel A, Regelson W, Kalimi M. Dehydroepiandrosterone protects hippocampal neurons against neurotoxin-induced cell death: mechanism of action. *Proc. Soc. Exp. Biol. Med.*, 1999, 222, 145-149.

Carpenter SS, Hatchett AD, Fuller MA. Catatonic schizophrenia and the use of memantine. *Ann. Pharmacother.*, 2006, 40, 344-6.

Charalampopoulos I, Tsatsanis C, Dermitzaki E, Alexaki VI, Castanas E, Margioris AN, Gravanis A. Dehydroepiandrosterone and allopregnanolone protect sympathoadrenal medulla cells against apoptosis via antiapoptotic Bcl-2 proteins. *Proc. Natl. Acad. Sci. USA,* 2004, 101, 8209-8214.

Chiang MY, Misner D, Kempermann G, Schikorski T, Giguere V, Sucov HM, Gage FH, Stevens CF, Evans RM. An essential role for retinoid receptors RARbeta and RXRgamma in long-term potentiation and depression. *Neuron*, 1998, 21,1353-1361.

Compagnone, N.A. and Mellon, S.H. Neurosteroids: biosynthesis and function of these novel neuromodulators. *Frontiers in Neuroendocrinology*, 2000, 21, 1-56.

Cooper R, Morre DJ, Morre DM. Medicinal benefits of green tea: Part I. Review of noncancer health benefits. *J. Altern. Complement Med.*, 2005, 11, 521-528.

Gallarda T, Loo H.Memantine (Ebixa): a new therapeutic strategy for the treatment of moderate to severe forms of Alzheimer's disease. *Encephale*, 2004, 30, 69-79.

Chavez-Noriega LE, Schaffhauser H, Campbell UC. Metabotropic glutamate receptors: potential drug targets for the treatment of schizophrenia. *Curr. Drug Targets CNS Neurol. Disord.*, 2002, 1, 261-281.

Chambon P: The retinoid signaling pathway: Molecular and genetic analyses. *Semin. Cell Biol.*, 1994, 5, 115-125.

Danysz W, Parsons CG. The NMDA receptor antagonist memantine as a symptomatological and neuroprotective treatment for Alzheimer's disease: preclinical evidence. *Int. J. Geriatr. Psychiatry*, 2003; 18 (suppl 1), 23-32.

Debonnel G, Bergeron R, de Montigny C. Potentiation by dehydroepiandrosterone of the neuronal response to N-methyl-D-aspartate in the CA3 region of the rat dorsal hippocampus: an effect mediated via sigma receptors. *J. Endocrinol.*, 1996, 150 (Suppl), 33-42.

Diamond DM, Branch BJ, Fleshner M.The neurosteroids dehydroepiandrosterone sulfate (DHEAS) enhances hippocampal primed burst, but not long-term potentiation. *Neuroscience Lett.*, 1996, 202, 204–208.

Dy, Grace K.; Adjei, Alex A. Novel Targets for Lung Cancer Therapy: Part I. *Journal of Clinical Oncology*, 2002, 20, 2881-2894.

Ehrenreich H, Siren AL. Neuroprotection--what does it mean?--What means do we have? *Eur. Arch Psychiatry Clin. Neurosci.*, 2001, 251, 149-151.

Ehrenreich H, Aust C, Krampe H, Jahn H, Jacob S, Herrmann M, Siren AL. Erythropoietin: novel approaches to neuroprotection in human brain disease. *Metab. Brain Dis.*, 2004, 19, 195-206.

Egashira N, Hayakawa K, Mishima K, Kimura H, Iwasaki K, Fujiwara M. Neuroprotective effect of gamma-glutamylethylamide (theanine) on cerebral infarction in mice. *Neurosci. Lett.*, 2004, 363, 58-61.

Ekborg-Ott KH, Taylor A, Armstrong DW. Varietal differences in the total and enantiomeric composition of theanine in tea. *J. Agric. Food Chem.*, 1997, 45, 353-363.

Esteva, Francisco J.; Glaspy, John; Baidas, Said; Laufman, Leslie; Hutchins, Laura; Dickler, Maura; Tripathy, Debu; Cohen, Roger; DeMichele, Angela; Yocum, Richard C.; Osborne, C. Kent; Hayes, Daniel F.; Hortobagyi, Gabriel N.; Winer, Eric; Demetri, George D. Multicenter Phase II Study of Oral Bexarotene for Patients With Metastatic Breast Cancer. *Journal of Clinical Oncology*, 2003, 21, 999-1006.

Fletcher EJ, MacDonald JF: Haloperidol interacts with the strychnine-insensitive glycine site at the NMDA receptor in cultured mouse hippocampal neurones. *Eur. J. Pharmacol.*, 1993, 235, 291-295.

Flood, J.F., Morley, J.E., Roberts, E. Memory-enhancing effects in male mice of Pregnenolone and steroids metabolically derived from it. *Proc. Natl. Acad. Sci.*, 1992, 89, 1567–1571.

Flood, J.F., Morley, J.E., Roberts, E. Pregnenolone sulfate enhances post-training memory processes when injected in very low doses into limbic system structures: the amygdala is by far the most sensitive. *Proc. Natl. Acad. Sci. USA*, 1995, 92, 10806–10810.

Friess E.,T. Schiffelholz,T. Steckler and A. Steiger. Dehydroepiandrosterone – a neurosteroids. *European Journal of Clinical Investigation*, 2000, 30 (Suppl. 3), 46–50.

Gambi F, De Berardis D, Sepede G, Quartesan R, Calcagni E, Salerno RM, Conti CM,
Ferro FM. Cannabinoid receptors and their relationships with neuropsychiatric disorders. *Int. J. Immunopathol. Pharmacol.*, 2005, 18, 15-19.

Gasior, M., Carter, R.B., Witkin, J.M. Neuroactive steroids: potential therapeutic use in neurological and psychiatric disorders. *Trends Pharmacol. Sci*, 1999, 20, 107–112.

George, M.S., Guidotti, A., Rubinow, D., Pan, P., Mikalauskas, K., Post, R.M. CSF neuroactive steroids in affective disorders: pregnenolone, progesterone and DBI. *Biol. Psychiatry*, 1994, 35, 775–780.

Goff, DC, Coyle, JT. The Emerging Role of Glutamate in the Pathophysiology and Treatment of Schizophrenia. *Am. J. Psychiatry,* 2001,158,1367-1377.

Goodyer IM, Park RJ, Netherton CM, Herbert J. Possible role of cortisol and dehydroepiandrosterone in human development and psychopathology. *British Journal of Psychiatry,* 2001,179, 243–249.

Gorgun G, Foss F. Immunomodulatory effects of RXR rexinoids: modulation of high-affinity IL-2R expression enhances susceptibility to denileukin diftitox. *Blood*, 2002,100, 1399-1403.

Goodman, A.B. Chromosomal locations and modes of action of genes of the retinoid (vitamin A) system support their involvement in the etiology of schizophrenia. *American Journal of Medical Genetics*, 1995, 60, 335-348.

Goodman, AB: Congenital anomalies of schizophrenic probands may indicate a retinoid pathology. *Schizophrenia Research*, 1996, 19, 163-170.

Goodman,AB.Three independent lines of evidence suggest retinoids as causal to schizophrenia. *Proc. Natl. Acad. Sci. USA*, 1998, 95, 7240-44.

Guazzo EP, Kirkpatrick PJ, Goodyer IM, Shiers HM, Herbert J. Cortisol, dehydroepiandrosterone (DHEA), and DHEA sulfate in the cerebrospinal fluid of man: relation to blood levels and the effects of age. *J. Clin. Endocrinol. Metab*., 1996, 81, 3951–3960.

Gursoy E, Cardounel A, Kalimi M. Pregnenolone protects mouse hippocampal (HT-22) cells against glutamate and amyloid beta protein toxicity. *Neurochem. Res*., 2001, 26, 15-21.

Hashimoto T, Bergen SE, Nguyen QL, et al. Relationship of brain-derived neurotrophic factor and its receptor TrkB to altered inhibitory prefrontal circuitry in schizophrenia. *J. Neurosci.*, 2005, 25, 372-383.

Heresco-Levy U, Javitt D, Ermilov M, Mordel C, Silipo G, Lichenstein M: Efficacy of high-dose glycine in the treatment of enduring negative symptoms of schizophrenia. *Arch Gen. Psychiatry*, 1999, 56, 29-36.

Heydari, B. and Le Melledo, J.M. Low pregnenolone sulphate plasma concentrations in patients with generalized social phobia. *Psychol. Med*., 2002, 32, 929-933.

Hong WK, Lippman SM, Itri LM, et al: Prevention of second primary tumors with isotretinoin in squamous-cell carcinoma of the head and neck. *N Engl. J. Med*, 1990, 323, 795-801.

Hu Y, Cardounel A, Gursoy E, Anderson P, Kalimi M. Anti-stress effects of dehydroepiandrosterone: protection of rats against repeated immobilization stress-induced weight loss, glucocorticoid receptor production, and lipid peroxidation. *Biochem. Pharmacol*., 2000, 59, 753-762.

Hurst RE. Bexarotene ligand pharmaceuticals. *Curr. Opin. Investig. Drugs*, 2000, 1, 514-523.

Ito K, Nagato Y, Aoi N, et al. Effects of L-theanine on the release of alpha-brain waves in human volunteers. Nippon Nogeikagaku Kaishi, 1998, 72, 153–157.

Jann MW. Implications for atypical antipsychotics in the treatment of schizophrenia: neurocognition effects and a neuroprotective hypothesis. *Pharmacotherapy,* 2004, 24,1759-1783.

Jarskog LF, Selinger ES, Lieberman JA, Gilmore JH. Apoptotic proteins in the temporal cortex in schizophrenia: high Bax/Bcl-2 ratio without caspase-3 activation. *Am. J. Psychiatry*, 2004, 161, 109-115.

Javitt DC, Zylberman I, Zukin SR, Heresco-Levy U, Lindenmayer JP. Amelioration of negative symptoms in schizophrenia by glycine. *Am. J. Psychiatry*, 1994, 151,1234-1236.

Juneja LR, Chu DC, Okubo T, Nagato Y, Yokogoshi H. L-theanine—a unique amino acid of green tea and its relaxation effect in humans. *Trends Food Sci. Technol.*,1999, 10,199-204.

Kakuda T. Neuroprotective effects of the green tea components theanine and catechins. *Biol. Pharm. Bull.*, 2002, 25, 1513-1518.

Kakuda T, Matsuura T, Sagesaka Y, Kawasaki T. Product and method for inhibiting caffeine stimulation with theanine. *US Patent* 5,501,866; 1996.

Kakuda T, Nozawa A, Unno T, Okamura N, Okai O. Inhibiting effects of theanine on caffeine stimulation evaluated by EEG in the rat. *Biosci. Biotechnol. Biochem.*, 2000, 64, 287-293.

Kakuda T, Nozawa A, Sugimoto A, Niino H. Inhibition by theanine of binding of [^{3}H] AMPA, [^{3}H] kainate, and [^{3}H]MDL 105,519 to glutamate receptors. *Biosci. Biotechnol. Biochem.*, 2002, 66, 2683-2686.

Kamath AB, Wang L, Das H, Li L, Reinhold VN, et al. Antigens in tea-beverage prime human γδ T cells *in vitro* and *in vivo* for memory and nonmemory antibacterial cytokine responses. *Proc. Natl. Acad. Sci. USA*, 2003,100, 6009-6014.

Karishma KK, Herbert J. Dehydroepiandrosterone (DHEA) stimulates neurogenesis in the hippocampus of the rat, promotes survival of newly formed neurons and prevents corticosterone-induced suppression. *Eur. J. Neurosci.,* 2002, 16, 445-453.

Kent JM, Mathew SJ, Gorman JM. Molecular targets in the treatment of anxiety. *Biol. Psychiatry*, 2002, 52,1008-1030.

Khuri FR, Rigas JR, Figlin RA, Gralla RJ, Shin DM, Munden R, Fox N, Huyghe MR Multi-institutional phase I/II trial of oral bexarotene in combination with cisplatin and vinorelbine in previously untreated patients with advanced non-small-cell lung cancer. *J. Clin. Oncol.*, 2001, 19, 2626-2637.

Kimonides VG, Khatibi NH, Svendsen CN, Sofroniew MV, Herbert J. Dehydroepiandrosterone (DHEA) and DHEA-sulfate (DHEAS) protect hippocampal neurons against excitatory amino acid-induced neurotoxicity. *Proc. Natl. Acad. Sci. USA,* 1998, 95, 1852-1857.

Kimonides VG, Spillantini MG, Sofroniew MV, Fawcett JW, Herbert J. Dehydroepiandrosterone antagonizes the neurotoxic effects of corticosterone and translocation of stress-activated protein kinase 3 in hippocampal primary cultures. *Neuroscience*, 1999, 89, 429-436.

Kimura R, Murata T. Influence of alkylamides of glutamic acid and related compounds on the central nervous system. I. Central depressant effect of theanine. *Chem. Pharm. Bull.* (Tokyo), 1971,19, 1257-1261.

Kimura R, Murata T. Effect of theanine on norepinephrine and serotonin levels in rat brain. *Chem. Pharm. Bull.* (Tokyo), 1986, 34, 3053-3057.

Kimura R, Murata T. Influence of alkylamides of glutamic acid and related compounds on the central nervous system. I. Central depressant effect of theanine. *Chem. Pharm. Bull.* (Tokyo), 1971, 19, 1257-12561.

Kitaoka S, Hayashi H, Yokogoshi H, Suzuki Y. Transmural potential changes associated with the *in vitro* absorption of theanine in the guinea pig intestine. *Biosci. Biotechnol. Biochem*., 1996, 60, 1768-17671.

Kito M, Kokura H, Izaki J, Sasaoka K. Theanine, a precursor of the phloroglucinol nucleus of catechins in the tea plants. *Phytochemistry*, 1968, 7, 599-603.

Knoll JL 4th, Garver DL, Ramberg JE, Kingsbury SJ, Croissant D, McDermott B. Heterogeneity of the psychoses: is there a neurodegenerative psychosis? *Schizophr. Bull*., 1998, 24, 365-379.

Kobayashi K, Nagato Y, Aoi N, Juneja LR, Kim M, et al. Effects of L-theanine on the release of α-brain waves in human volunteers. Nippon Nogeikagaku Kaishi, 1998, 72, 153-157.

Krebs M, Leopold K, Hinzpeter A, Schaefer M. Neuroprotective agents in schizophrenia and affective disorders. *Expert Opin. Pharmacother*., 2006, 7, 837-848.

Krezel W, Ghyselinck N, Samad TA, Dupe V, Kastner P, Borrelli E, Chambon P Impaired locomotion and dopamine signaling in retinoid receptor mutant mice. *Science,* 1998, 279, 863-867.

Kurata K, Takebayashi M, Morinobu S, Yamawaki S. Beta-estradiol, dehydroepiandrosterone, and dehydroepiandrosterone sulfate protect against N-methyl-D-aspartate-induced neurotoxicity in rat hippocampal neurons by different mechanisms. *J Pharmacol. Exp. Ther.,* 2004, 311, 237-245.

Lang UE, Jockers-Scherubl MC, Hellweg R. State of the art of the neurotrophin hypothesis in psychiatric disorders: implications and limitations. *J. Neural. Transm.,* 2004, 111, 387-411.

Lapchak PA, Araujo DM. Preclinical development of neurosteroids as neuroprotective agents for the treatment of neurodegenerative diseases. *Int. Rev. Neurobiol*., 2001, 46, 379-397.

Le Goascogne, C., Robel, P., Gouezou, M., Sananes, N., Baulieu, E-E. and Waterman, M. Neurosteroids: cytochrome P-450scc in rat brain. *Science*, 1987, 237, 1212-1215.

Leid M, Kastner P, Chambon P: Multiplicity generates diversity in the retinoic acid signaling pathways. *Trends Biochem. Sci,* 1992, 17, 427-433.

Lewis DA, Levitt P. Schizophrenia as a disorder of neurodevelopment. *Annu. Rev. Neurosci*., 2002, 25, 409-432.

Lhullier FL, Nicolaidis R, Riera NG, Cipriani F, Junqueira D, Dahm KC, Brusque AM, Souza DO. Dehydroepiandrosterone increases synaptosomal glutamate release and improves the performance in inhibitory avoidance task. *Pharmacol. Biochem. Behav.,* 2004, 77, 601-606.

Lidsky TI, Yablonsky-Alter E, Zuck LG, Banerjee SP: Antipsychotic drug effects on glutamatergic activity. *Brain Res.,* 1997, 764, 46-52.

Lu K, Gray MA, Oliver C, Liley DT, Harrison BJ, Bartholomeusz CF, Phan KL,Nathan PJ.The acute effects of L-theanine in comparison with alprazolam on anticipatory nxiety in humans. *Hum. Psychopharmacol*., 2004, 19, 457-465.

McGavack, T.H., Chevalley, J., Weissberg, J. The use of delta-5-pregnenolone in various clinical disorders. *J. Clin. Endocrinol.,* 1951, 11, 559–577.

McCoy L, Richfield EK: Chronic antipsychotic treatment alters glycine-stimulated NMDA receptor binding in rat brain. *Neurosci. Lett.,* 1996, 213, 137-141 .

Mahadik SP, Evans D, Lal H. Oxidative stress and role of antioxidant and omega-3 essential fatty acid supplementation in schizophrenia. *Prog. Neuropsychopharmacol. Biol. Psychiatry*, 2001, 25, 463-493.

Manji HK, Moore GJ, Chen G. Lithium at 50: have the neuroprotective effects of this unique cation been overlooked? *Biol. Psychiatry*, 1999, 46, 929-940.

Majewska MD, Demirgoren S, Spivak CE, London ED. The neurosteroid dehydroepiandrosterone sulfate is an antagonist of the GABA-A receptor. *Brain Res.*, 1990, 526, 143–146.

Majewska MD. Neurosteroids: endogenous bimodal modulators of the GABAA receptor. Mechanism of action and physiological significance. Prog Neurobiol., 1992, 38, 379-395.

Majewska MD. Neuronal actions of dehydroepiandrosterone. Possible roles in brain development, aging, memory, and affect. *Ann. N Y Acad. Sci.*, 1995, 774,111-120.

Mao X, Barger SW. Neuroprotection by dehydroepiandrosterone-sulfate: role of an NFkappaB-like factor. *Neuroreport.,* 1998, 9, 759-763.

Martin S, Bradley J, Cotter T: HL-60 cells induced to differentiate towards neutrophils subsequently die via apoptosis. *Clin. Exp. Immunol.,* 1990, 79, 448-453.

Marx CE, Stevens RD, Shampine LJ, Uzunova V, Trost WT, Butterfield MI, Massing MW, Hamer RM, Morrow AL, Lieberman JA. Neuroactive steroids are altered in schizophrenia and bipolar disorder: relevance to pathophysiology and therapeutics. *Neuropsychopharmacology*, 2006, 31, 1249-1263.

Mason R. 200 mg of Zen; L-theanine boosts alpha waves, promotes alert relaxation. *Alternative and Complementary Therapies*, 2001, 7, 91-95.

Mayo, W., Le Moal, M. and Abrous, D.N. Pregnenolone sulfate and aging of cognitive functions: behavioral, neurochemical, and morphological investigations. *Hormonal Behav.*, 2001, 40, 215-217.

McCaffery P, Drager DC. High levels of a retinoic acid-generating dehydrogenase in the meso telencephalic dopamine system. *Proceedings of the National Academy of Sciences* (USA), 1994, 91, 7772-7776.

McGlashan TH, Hoffman RE. Schizophrenia as a disorder of developmentally reduced synaptic connectivity. *Arch Gen. Psychiatry,* 2000, 57, 637-648.

Meador-Woodruff JH, Healy DJ: Glutamate receptor expression in schizophrenic brain. Brain *Res. Brain Res. Rev.,* 2000, 31, 288-294.

Meieran SE, Reus VI, Webster R, Shafton R, Wolkowitz OM. Chronic pregnenolone effects in normal humans: attenuation of benzodiazepine-induced sedation. *Psychoneuroendocrinology,* 2004, 29, 486-500.

Melchior, C.L., Ritzmann, R.F. Pregnenolone and pregnenolone sulfate, alone and with ethanol, in mice on the plus-maze. *Pharmacol. Biochem. Behav.*, 1994, 48, 893–897.

Middleton FA, Mirnics K, Pierri JN, Lewis DA, Levitt P. Gene expression profiling reveals alterations of specific metabolic pathways in schizophrenia. *J. Neurosci.*, 2002, 22, 2718-2729.

Migues PV, Johnston AN, Rose SP. Dehydroepiandosterone and its sulphate enhance memory retention in day-old chicks. *Neuroscience,* 2002, 109, 243-251.

Miguel-Hidalgo JJ, Alvarez XA, Cacabelos R, Quack G. Neuroprotection by memantine against neurodegeneration induced by beta-amyloid(1-40). *Brain Res.*, 2002, 958, 210-221.

Millan MJ. The neurobiology and control of anxious states. *Prog. Neurobiol.*, 2003, 70, 83–244.

Misner DL, Jacobs S, Shimizu Y, de Urquiza AM, Solomin L, Perlmann T, De Luca LM, Stevens CF, Evans RM. Vitamin A deprivation results in reversible loss of hippocampal long-term synaptic plasticity. *Proc. Natl. Acad. Sci. USA*, 2001, 98, 11714-11719.

Moises HW, Zoega T, Gottesman II. The glial growth factors deficiency and synaptic destabilization hypothesis of schizophrenia. *BMC Psychiatry*, 2002, 3, 2:8.

Murray RM. Neurodevelopmental schizophrenia: the rediscovery of dementia praecox. *Br. J. Psychiatry Suppl.*, 1994, 25, 6-12.

Nachshoni T, Ebert T, Abramovitch Y, Assael-Amir M, Kotler M, Maayan R, Weizman A, Strous RD.Improvement of extrapyramidal symptoms following dehydroepiandrosterone (DHEA) administration in antipsychotic treated schizophrenia patients: a randomized, double-blind placebo controlled trial. *Schizophr. Res.*, 2005, 79, 251-256.

Nafziger AN, Bowlin SJ, Jenkins PL, et al: Longitudinal changes in dehydroepiandrosterone concentrations in men and women. *J. Lab. Clin. Med.*, 1998, 131, 316–323.

Nagasawa K, Aoki H, Yasuda E, Nagai K, Shimohama S, Fujimoto S. Possible involvement of group I mGluRs in neuroprotective effect of theanine. *Biochem. Biophys. Res. Commun.*, 2004, 320, 116-122.

Neeman G, Blanaru M, Bloch B, Kremer I, Ermilov M, Javitt DC, Heresco-Levy U. Relation of plasma glycine, serine, and homocysteine levels to schizophrenia symptoms and medication type. *Am. J. Psychiatry*, 2005, 162,1738-1740.

Nozawa A, Umezawa K, Kobayashi K, Kawahara M, Muramoto K, et al. Theanine, a major flavorous amino acid in green tea leaves, inhibits glutamate-induced neurotoxicity on cultured rat cerebral cortical neurons. *Soc. Neurosci. Abstr.*, 1998, 24(382.6).

Okubo T, Ozeki M, Inden T, Juneja LR, Hisanabe M, et al. Compositions for regulating desire for smoking. *US Patent Application,* 2003/003130; Jan. 2, 2003.

Orgogozo JM, Rigaud AS, Stoffler A, Mobius HJ, Forette F. Efficacy and safety of memantine in patients with mild–moderate vascular dementia: a randomized, placebo controlled trial (MMM 300). *Stroke*, 2002, 33,1834-1839.

Oridate N, Lotan D, Xu XC, et al: Differential induction of apoptosis by all-trans-retinoic acid and N-(4-hydroxyphenyl)retinamide in human head and neck squamous cell carcinoma cell lines. *Clin. Cancer Res.,* 1996, 2, 855-863.

Ozeki M, Yao H, Okubo T, Juneja LR. Compositions for promoting sleep. US Patent Application 2002/0188025, 2002.

Querfeld C, Nagelli LV, Rosen ST, Kuzel TM, Guitart J. Bexarotene in the treatment of cutaneous T-cell lymphoma. *Expert Opin. Pharmacother.,* 2006, 7, 907-915.

Piketty C, Jayle D, Leplege A, Castiel P, Ecosse E, Gonzalez-Canali G, Sabatier B, Boulle N, Debuire B, Le Bouc Y, Baulieu EE, Kazatchkine MD. Double-blind placebo-controlled trial of oral dehydroepiandrosterone in patients with advanced HIV disease. *Clin. Endocrinol.* (Oxf)., 2001, 55, 325-330.

Pincus, G., Hoagland, H.Effects of administered pregnenolone on fatiguing psychomotor performance. *J. Aviation Med.,* 1944, 15, 98–115.

Pincus, G., Hoagland, H. Effects on industrial production of the administration of Pregnenolone to factory workers, I. *Psychosom. Med.*, 1945, 7, 342–346.

Pisu MG, Serra M. Neurosteroids and neuroactive drugs in mental disorders. *Life Sci.*, 2004, 74, 3181-3197.

Potyk, D. Treatments for Alzheimer disease. *South Med. J.* 2005 Jun;98(6):628-35.

Racchi M, Balduzzi C, Corsini E. Dehydroepiandrosterone (DHEA) and the aging brain: flipping a coin in the "fountain of youth". *CNS Drug Rev.*, 2003, 9, 21-40.

Rapoport JL, Addington AM, Frangou S, Psych MR. The neurodevelopmental model of schizophrenia: update 2005. *Mol. Psychiatry*, 2005, 10, 434-449.

Rasmusson AM, Vythilingam M, Morgan CA 3rd. The neuroendocrinology of posttraumatic stress disorder: new directions. *CNS Spectr.*, 2003, 8, 651-656, 665-667.

Reddy, D.S., Kaur, G., Kulkarni, S.K. Sigma (sigma1) receptor mediated anti-depressant-like effects of neurosteroids in the Porsolt forced swim test. *Neuroreport.,* 1998, 9, 3069–3073.

Reisberg B, Doody R, Stoffler A, et al. Memantine in moderate-tosevere Alzheimer disease. *NEJM,* 2003, 348, 1333–1341.

Rigas JR , Maurer LH, Meyer LP, Hammond SM, Crisp MR, Parker BA, Truglia JA. Targretin, a selective retinoid X receptor ligand (LGD1069), vinorelbine and cisplatin for the treatment of non-small cell lung cancer (NSCLC): a phase I/II trial. *Proc. Annu. Meet Am. Soc. Clin. Oncol.*, 1997,16, A1724.

Ritsner MS, Maayan R, Gibel A, Weizman A. Low serum pregnenolone levels are associated with trait-anxiety, but not with clinical symptomatology among chronic treated patients with schizophrenia. *European Neuropsychopharmacology*, 2006a, in press.

Ritsner, MS, Gibel, A., Ratner, Y., Tsinovoy, G., Strous, D. Improvement of sustained attention, visual and movement skills, but not clinical symptomatology, following dehydroepiandrosterone augmentation in schizophrenia: a randomized double-blind, placebo-controlled, crossover trial. *Int. Clin. Psychopharmacol.*, 2006b (in press).

Roberts, E., Fitten, L.J. Serum steroid levels in two old men with Alzheimer's disease (AD) before and after oral administration of dehydroepiandrosterone (DHEA). Pregnenolone synthesis may be ratelimiting in aging. In: Kalimi, M., Regelson, W. (Eds.), The Biological Role of Dehydroepiandrosterone (DHEA). de Gruyter, Berlin, 1990, 43–63.

Rogawski MA, Wenk GL. The neuropharmacological basis for the use of memantine in the treatment of Alzheimer's disease. *CNS Drug Rev.,* 2003, 9, 275-308.

Rogawski MA, What is the rationale for new treatment strategies in Alzheimer's disease? *CNS Spectr.*, 2004, 9(7 Suppl 5), 6-12.

Roozendaal B, McGaugh JL.Amygdaloid nuclei lesions differentially affect glucocorticoid-induced memory enhancement in an inhibitory avoidance task. *Neurobiol. Learn Mem.*, 1996, 65, 1–8.

Rupprecht, R. The neuropsychopharmacological potential of neuroactive steroids. *J. Psychiatr. Res.*, 1997, 31, 297–314.

Sadzuka Y, Sugiyama T, Miyagishima A, Nozawa Y, Hirota S. The effects of theanine, as a novel biochemical modulator, on the antitumor activity of adriamycin. *Cancer Lett.*, 1996, 105, 203-209.

Sadzuka Y, Sugiyama T, Sonobe T. Improvement of idarubicin induced antitumor activity and bone marrow suppression by theanine, a component of tea. *Cancer Lett.*, 2000, 158,119-124.

Sadzuka Y, Sugiyama T, Suzuki T, Sonobe T. Enhancement of the activity of doxorubicin by inhibition of glutamate transporter. *Toxicol. Lett.*, 2001, 123,159-167.

Sadzuka Y, Yamashita Y, Kishimoto S, Fukushima S, Takeuchi Y, et al. Glutamate transporter mediated increase of antitumor activity by theanine, an amino acid in green tea [in Japanese]. Yakugaku Zasshi., 2002, 122, 995-999.

Sadzuka Y, Sugiyama T, Nagamine M, Umegaki K, Sonobe T. Efficacy of theanine is connected with theanine metabolism by any enzyme, not only drug metabolizing enzymes. *Food Chem. Toxicol.*, 2006, 44, 286-292.

Sakato Y. The chemical constituents of tea: III. A new amide theanine. Nippon Nogeikagaku Kaishi, 1949, 23, 262-267.

Samad T A, Krezel W, Chambron P, Borrelli E. Regulation of dopaminergic pathways by retinoids: activation of the D2 receptor promoter by members of the retinoic acid receptor-retinoid X receptor family. *Proceedings of the National Academy of Sciences* (USA), 1997, 94, 14349-14354.

Satre MA, Ugen KE, Kochhar DM. Developmental changes in endogenous retinoids during pregnancy and embryogenesis in the mouse. *Biology of Reproduction*, 1992, 46, 802-810.

Schmidt WJ, Kretschmer BD. Behavioural pharmacology of glutamate receptors in the basal ganglia. *Neurosci. Biobehav. Rev.*, 1997, 21, 381-392.

Schmidt PJ, Daly RC, Bloch M, Smith MJ, Danaceau MA, St Clair LS, Murphy JH, Haq N, Rubinow DR. Dehydroepiandrosterone monotherapy in midlife-onset major and minor depression. *Arch Gen. Psychiatry*, 2005, 62, 154-162.

Shenton ME, Dickey CC, Frumin M, McCarley RW. A review of MRI findings in schizophrenia. *Schizophr. Res.*, 2001, 49, 1-52.

Sherman SI. Etiology, diagnosis, and treatment recommendations for central hypothyroidism associated with bexarotene therapy for cutaneous T-cell lymphoma. *Clin. Lymphoma*, 2003, 3, 249-252.

Semeniuk, T., Jhangri, G., Le Melledo, J. Neuroactive steroid levels in patients with generalized anxiety disorder. *J. Neuropsychiatry Clin. Neurosci.*, 2001, 13, 396–398.

Shalita, A.R. Mucocutaneous and systemic toxicity of retinoids: monitoring and management. *Dermatologica*, 1987, 1, 151-157.

Sleeper, RB. Antipsychotic dose-sparing effect with addition of memantine. *Ann. Pharmacother.*, 2005, 39, 1573-1576.

Smit JV, De Jong EM, Van De Kerkhof PC. Effects of Oral Bexarotene (Targretin) on the Minimal Erythema Dose for Broadspectrum UVB Light. *Skin Pharmacol. Appl. Skin Physiol.*, 2003, 16, 237-241.

Sporn M, Roberts A: Role of retinoids in differentiation and carcinogenesis. *J. Natl. Cancer Inst.*, 1984, 73, 1381-1387.

Stark AK, Uylings HB, Sanz-Arigita E, Pakkenberg B. Glial cell loss in the anterior cingulate cortex, a subregion of the prefrontal cortex, in subjects with schizophrenia. *Am. J. Psychiatry,* 2004, 161, 882-888.

Stoffel-Wagner B. Neurosteroid metabolism in the human brain. *Eur. J. Endocrinol.*, 2001, 145, 669-679.

Stoffel-Wagner, B. Neurosteroid biosynthesis in the human brain and its clinical implications. *Ann. N. Y. Acad. Sci.,* 2003, 1007, 64-78.

Strous RD, Maayan R, Lapidus R, Stryjer R, Lustig M, Kotler M, Weizman A. Dehydroepiandrosterone augmentation in the management of negative, depressive, and anxiety symptoms in schizophrenia. *Arch Gen. Psychiatry*, 2003, 60, 133-141.

Sugiyama T, Sadzuka Y. Theanine, a specific glutamate derivative in green tea, reduces the adverse reactions of doxorubicin by changing the glutathione level. *Cancer Lett.*, 2004, 212, 177-184.

Tagawa, N., Tamanaka, J., Fujinami, A., Kobayashi, Y., Takano, T., Fukata, S., Kuma, K., Tada, H. and Amino, N. Serum dehydroepiandrosterone, dehydropiandrosterone sulfate, and pregnonolone sulfate concentrations in patients with hyperthyroidism and hypothyroidism. *Clin. Chem*., 2000, 46, 523-528.

Takahashi H, Nakajima A, Sekihara H.Dehydroepiandrosterone (DHEA) and its sulfate (DHEAS) inhibit the apoptosis in human peripheral blood lymphocytes. *J. Steroid Biochem. Mol. Biol.*, 2004, 88, 261-264.

Tariot PN, Farlow MR, Grossberg GT, Graham SM, McDonald S, Gergel I, for the Memantine Study Group. Memantine treatment in patients with moderate to severe Alzheimer's disease already receiving donepezil: a randomized controlled trial. *JAMA*, 2004, 291, 317-324.

Terashima T, Takido J, Yokogoshi H. Time-dependent changes of amino acids in the serum, liver, brain and urine of rats administered with theanine. *Biosci. Biotechnol. Biochem.,* 1999, 63, 615-618.

Thomas, C. Memantine and Catatonic Schizophrenia. *Am. J. Psychiatry*, 2005, 162, 626.

Tsuge H, Sano S, Hayakawa T, Kakuda T, Unno T. Theanine, γ-glutamylethylamide, is metabolized by renal phosphate-independent glutaminase. *Biochim. Biophys. Acta*, 2003, 1620, 47-53.

Tsutsui K, Matsunaga M, Miyabara H, Ukena K. Neurosteroid biosynthesis in the quail brain: a review. *J. Exp. Zoolog. A Comp. Exp. Biol.,* 2006, 305, 733-742.

Ueda T, Nagato Y, Tanaka Y, Okubo T, Kobayashi K, et al. Composition comprising theanine. US Patent 6, 589, 566; July 8, 2003.

Unno T, Suzuki Y, Kakuda T, Hayakawa T, Tsuge H. Metabolism of theanine, γ-glutamylethylamide, in rats. *J. Agric. Food Chem*., 1999, 47,1593-1596.

Yokogoshi H, Kato Y, Sagesaka YM, Takihara-Matsuura T, Kakuda T, et al. Reduction effect of theanine on blood pressure and brain 5-hydroxyindoles in spontaneously hypertensive rats. *Biosci. Biotechnol. Biochem.,* 1995, 59, 615-618.

Yokozawa T, Dong E. Influence of green tea and its three major components upon lowdensity lipoprotein oxidation. *Exp. Toxicol. Pathol.,* 1997, 49, 329-335.

Yokogoshi H, Kobayashi M, Mochizuki M, Terashima T. Effect of theanine, r-glutamylethylamide, on brain monoamines and striatal dopamine release in conscious rats. *Neurochem. Res*., 1998a, 3, 667–673.

Yokogoshi H, Mochizuki M, Saitoh K. Theanine-induced reduction of brain serotonin concentration in rats. *Biosci. Biotech. Biochem*., 1998b, 62, 816–817.

Yokogoshi H, Kobayashi M. Hypotensive effect of gamma-glutamylmethylamide in spontaneously hypertensive rats. *Life Sci*., 1998c, 62, 1065-1068.

van Vollenhoven RF. Dehydroepiandrosterone for the treatment of systemic lupus erythematosus. *Expert Opin. Pharmacother.,* 2002, 3, 23-31.

Veiga S, Garcia-Segura LM, Azcoitia I. Neuroprotection by the steroids pregnenolone and dehydroepiandrosterone is mediated by the enzyme aromatase. *J. Neurobiol*., 2003, 56, 398-406.

Wagner E, Luo T, Drager UC. Retinoic acid synthesis in the postnatal mouse brain marks distinct developmental stages and functional systems. *Cereb. Cortex*., 2002,12, 1244-1253.

Wen S, Dong K, Onolfo JP, Vincens M. Treatment with dehydroepiandrosterone sulfate increases NMDA receptors in hippocampus and cortex. *Eur. J. Pharmacol.*, 2001, 430, 373-374.

Wenk GL, Danysz W, Mobley SL. MK-801, memantine and amantadine show neuroprotective activity in the nucleus basalis magnocellularis. *Eur. J. Pharmacol. Environ. Toxicol.*, 1995, 293, 267-270.

Wenk GL. Neuropathologic changes in Alzheimer's disease: potential targets for treatment. *J. Clin. Psychiatry*, 2006, 67 (Suppl 3), 3-7.

Widstrom RL, Dillon JS. Is there a receptor for dehydroepiandrosterone or dehydroepiandrosterone sulfate? *Semin. Reprod. Med.*, 2004, 22, 289-298.

Winblad B, Poritis N. Memantine in severe dementia: results of the 9M-Best Study (Benefit and efficacy in severely demented patients during treatment with memantine). *Int. J. Geriatr. Pysch.*, 1999, 14, 135–146.

Wolf OT, Kirschbaum C. Actions of dehydroepiandrosterone and its sulfate in the central nervous system:effects on cognition and emotion in animals and humans. *Brain Res. Brain Res. Rev.*, 1999, 30, 264-288.

Wolkowitz OM, Reus VI, Roberts E, Manfredi F, Chan T, Raum WJ, Ormiston S, Johnson R, Canick J, Brizendine L, Weingartner H. Dehydroepiandrosterone (DHEA) treatment of depression. *Biol. Psychiatry,* 1997, 41, 311-318.

Wolkowitz OM, Reus VI, Keebler A, Nelson N, Friedland M, Brizendine L, Roberts E. Double-blind treatment of major depression with dehydroepiandrosterone. *Am. J. Psychiatry,* 1999, 156, 646-649.

Wood PL. The NMDA receptor complex: a long and winding road to therapeutics. *Idrugs,* 2005, 8, 229-235.

Zheng G, Sayama K, Okubo T, Juneja LR, Oguni I. Anti-obesity effects of three major components of green tea, catechins, caffeine and theanine, in mice. *In Vivo*, 2004, 18, 55-62.

Zwain IH, Yen SS. Neurosteroidogenesis in astrocytes, oligodendrocytes, and neurons of cerebral cortex of rat brain. *Endocrinology*, 1999, 140, 3843-3852.

In: New Hope for Mental Disturbances
Editors: Vladimir Lerner and Chanoch Meodownik
ISBN 978-1-60692-691-8

Chapter 8

MELATONIN AND SCHIZOPHRENIA

Yoram Barak[1]* and Dov Aizenberg[2]
1. Sackler Faculty of Medicine, Tel-Aviv University
and Psychogeriatric Department at the Abarbanel Mental Health Cente, Israel
2. Geha Mental Health Center affiliated with the Sackler Faculty of Medicine,
Tel-Aviv University, Israel.

ABSTRACT

In recent years the spectrum of known effects of melatonin was reported to exceed by far the original discoveries. Melatonin regulates, circadian and seasonal rhythms, such as the sleep-wake cycle and acts as an immunostimulator and cytoprotective agent. The association between melatonin and schizophrenia has been studied in several clinical domains such as sleep, cognition and tardive dyskinesia. The presumed pathophysiology and mechanism is thought to be related to the regulation of central dopaminergic pathways. In addition, recent clinical and research data indicates that melatonin may be advantageous as a complementary intervention for sleep disturbances of schizophrenia patients and possibly for patients suffering from tardive dyskinesia.

INTRODUCTION

The use of complementary medicines for subjects with mental health problems is documented and probably widespread. As their effectiveness is often not established and they may have significant adverse and side effects Werneke and colleagues have recently reviewed complementary medicines routinely used by health care professionals [1]. They concluded that potentially useful substances include ginkgo biloba and hydergine as cognitive enhancers, passion flower and valerian as sedatives, St John's Wort and s-adenosylmethionine as antidepressants, and selenium and folate to complement antidepressants. The evidence was

* Corresponding author: Yoram Barak, Sackler Faculty of Medicine, Tel-Aviv University and Psychogeriatric Department at the Abarbanel Mental Health Center. Mail address: 15 KKL Street, Bat-Yam, 59100, Israel. Tel: +972 3 5552738; Fax: +972 3 555 2738 :E-mail: mdybarak@netvision.net.il.

found to be less conclusive for the use of omega-3 fatty acids as augmentation treatment in schizophrenia and melatonin for tardive dyskinesia.

The melanophore contracting hormone melatonin was originally discovered as a skin-lightening molecule acting on frog and fish melanocytes [2]. Subsequently, melatonin was found to be present in all vertebrates, rhythmically secreted by the pineal gland, and involved in regulation of circadian and, sometimes, seasonal rhythms [3]. In recent years the spectrum of known effects of melatonin was reported to exceed by far the original discoveries. Melatonin regulates, circadian and seasonal rhythms, such as the sleep-wake cycle and acts as an immunostimulator and cytoprotective agent [4].

Light Effects on the Brain (adapted from Snyder et al, [5]). Circadian rhythms in the pineal gland were first observed by Wilbur Quay in 1963 and established as "true" rhythms that are maintained during dark periods, but dramatically modulated by light. Serotonin levels vary diurnally and inversely with melatonin. The biochemical link between serotonin and melatonin includes two converting enzymes the first acetylating serotonin to form *N*-acetyl serotonin and the second methylating *N*-acetyl serotonin to melatonin. The mechanisms underlying this process have been characterized as the following: nighttime release of noradrenaline in the pineal gland up-regulates the activity of 5-HT *N*-acetyltransferase and thus increases melatonin levels in a circadian fashion. A second essential property of nighttime melatonin synthesis by the pineal gland is its sensitivity to the length of night, conveying not only the day/night transition but also seasonal information. Adaptation of the organism to a changing environment, mediated in part by these processes, is an essential feature of physiological regulation. Translating the day/night rhythm into hormonal oscillations governs human and animal metabolism. Melatonin is rhythmically synthesized in response to signals from the biological clock located in the thalamic suprachiasmatic nucleus. The effects of altering the light/dark cycle, especially during seasons of long darkness with the goal of altering mood, are thought to be mediated to some degree by these molecular mechanisms.

Schizophrenia is a mental illness and one of the world's top ten causes of long-term medical disability. It is a life-long disorder requiring substantial care and great advances have been made in pharmacological and psychosocial treatment so that many patients can now live rewarding and meaningful lives in the community. The symptoms of schizophrenia vary but often include psychosis, apathy and withdrawal, and cognitive impairment leading to impairment in social and occupational functioning, and neglect in self-care. About 1% of the population is affected by schizophrenia, with similar rates across different regions, ethnic groups and sexes. The illness tends to be diagnosed between the ages of 16 and 45 years, and persists throughout the patient's lifetime. The course of schizophrenia may be understood with the stress-vulnerability model as the infrastructure. According to this model, schizophrenia is caused by an underlying psychobiological vulnerability, determined early in life by genetic and early developmental adverse effects. Once the vulnerability has been established, the onset of the illness and its course, including relapses, is determined by the complex dynamic interplay of biological and psychosocial factors. Among the severe psychiatric disorders, schizophrenia is the most disabling and requires a disproportionately high share of mental health services. The total direct and indirect costs of treating schizophrenia are high, estimated to be over 50 billion US$ in the USA and are correspondingly high in the UK and in Canada [6].

The cause of schizophrenia is unknown, but evidence suggests that genetic factors, familial loading, early environmental insults and social factors all contribute to its' emergence. To date no biological alterations that are pathognomonic of schizophrenia have been identified, although several pathophysiological differences exist in a wide range of brain structures often reflected in the dopaminergic and glutamatergic systems. Among the biological factors that affect the course of schizophrenia, medication, emotional expressivity within families and substance abuse are the most critical. Accordingly, the development of pharmacological interventions in schizophrenia has followed the knowledge gathered mainly in the domain of neurotransmitters. Antipsychotic medications can reduce severity of positive and negative symptoms and may even reduce susceptibility to relapses, whereas substance abuse can worsen symptoms and contribute to relapses. Novel interventions relying on data glimpsed from immunological and neuroendocrinological sources may be explored in the next decade. One of the compounds involved in this context is melatonin.

Melatonin and Schizophrenia

Nearly fifty years ago Altschule observed that intravenous administration of melatonin to schizophrenic patients in remission causes a worsening of psychotic symptoms which persists even after the treatment is interrupted [7]. This is probably the first report to associate melatonin with a psychotic condition. However, despite some studies in the decades since, only the persistent emphasis by Sandyk in the early 1990's significantly increased awareness of researchers as to the possible association between melatonin, tardive dyskinesia and schizophrenia [8, 9]. Sandyk had demonstrated that abnormal melatonin functions may be implicated in the pathophysiology of schizophrenia. He investigated chronic institutionalized schizophrenia patients showing that in patients with gradual onset schizophrenia had pineal calcification size that was significantly larger than those with sudden onset suggesting that the nature of onset of schizophrenia may be influenced by the activity of the pineal gland [10].

The hypothesis of an involvement of melatonin in schizophrenia received further support in studies adding data and understanding from various sources (for a brief review see Pacchierotti et al, [11]). First, melatonin has a structural similarity to some hallucinogenic substances (e.g., harmine, bufotenine, and psilocybin). Harmine cocaine and amphetamine induce the activation of the enzyme hydroxy-*O*-methyltransferase, which controls melatonin synthesis in the pineal gland [12, 13]. Furthermore, agents which produce symptoms closely resembling schizophrenic psychosis (cocaine, L-dopa, and amphetamine) also increase melatonin production. Research into the assimilation of LSD in monkey brains reveal a propensity for LSD concentrations in the pineal and pituitary glands, these accumulations being 7-8 times those found in the cerebral cortex [14].

The information available concerning circadian rhythms of melatonin in schizophrenia yields contradictory results [15]. Vigano et al [16] studied the behavior of melatonin secretion in schizophrenia patients versus healthy subjects. Light/dark rhythm of melatonin secretion showed physiological nocturnal increase in some patients, whereas the others showed an abnormally low melatonin peak during the night. Moreover, both light and night mean levels of melatonin were significantly lower in patients than in controls. This study would suggest that schizophrenia may be associated with diminished secretion of melatonin from the pineal gland, and pineal deficiency would be more evident in the chronic disease.

The biosynthetic activity of the pineal gland may be impaired in chronic schizophrenia and clinical improvement achieved by antipsychotic drugs does not induce changes in the production of melatonin. One of the important studies in this respect was completed by Rao et al [17] indicating a significant phase-advance of tryptophan, prolactin, and melatonin concentrations in the blood of more than 100 drug-free as well as treated schizophrenia patients. Recently, Schwartz and Erk [18] looked closely at the central D_2 dopamine receptor subtype involved in the pathogenesis and treatment of schizophrenia. Central D_2 receptors are also involved in thermoregulation via a CNS thermostat that governs the magnitude of core body thermoregulatory responses in proportion to amount of nocturnal melatonin secreted. They concluded that D_2 receptor-mediated hypothermia, an index of central D_2 receptor sensitivity, is regulated by the CNS thermostat in humans and that the abnormal D_2 receptors function in widely reported schizophrenia could be related to dysfunction of this thermostat thus suggesting the intermediary involvement of melatonin.

Seasonality of births of schizophrenia patients and seasonality of suicides have both been mentioned as possibly reflecting an association to melatonin secretion. Suicide is a major cause of death amongst schizophrenia patients. Suicides peak in May and June in the Northern Hemisphere and in November and December in the Southern Hemisphere. The risk increases between 8 and 50 percent in 20 countries surveyed. The author concluded that:" sunlight affects suicide risk through hormonal factors like melatonin" [19]. There is also a seasonal pattern in the births of schizophrenia patients. Studies confirm a 10 percent increase in these births in the Northern Hemisphere between February and April. This trend, coupled with findings that children of dark-skinned immigrants to northern countries have high rates of schizophrenia, led scientists to surmise a shortage of sunlight as a possible factor in the illness [19].

Treatment

Melatonin has been tested as a possible treatment for three conditions associated with schizophrenia: tardive dyskinesia (TD), cognitive dysfunction and sleep disturbances.

Tardive Dyskinesia

Attempts have been made to treat tardive dyskinesia with various antioxidants, mainly vitamin E. This treatment approach strategy relies on the assumption that tardive dyskinesia does not only result from supersensitivity of the dopamine receptor but is also related to the oxidative damage inflicted on basal structures by exposure to antipsychotic drugs [20, 21]. Meta-analysis of several trials of relatively small sample size has indicated that vitamin E protects against deterioration of tardive and may even improve the condition somewhat [22].

Melatonin is estimated to be about 10 times as powerful an antioxidant as vitamin E, in addition to its' attenuation of dopaminergic activity in the striatum and the hypothalamus [20, 21]. However, to date there have been only a few clinical trials demonstrating inconclusive results [21, 23], and thus larger prospective and well controlled trials are required to test its therapeutic effectiveness.

Shamir and colleagues [21, 23] attempted to assess the treatment effective of melatonin for tardive dyskinesia. In the first study [23] a group of 19 elderly patients aged 65 years or older suffering from chronic schizophrenia were randomly assigned in a double-blind, placebo-controlled, crossover trial to receive slow-release melatonin, 2 mg/day, or placebo for 4 weeks. Between treatments the patients underwent a 2-week washout period and were than switched to the other treatment arm for an additional 4 weeks. The Abnormal Involuntary Movement Scale (AIMS) was administered at baseline, 4 weeks, 6 weeks, and 10 weeks. Regular administration of antipsychotic and other medications was kept unchanged throughout the study. Following completion of the study by all participants the mean AIMS scores did not change significantly from baseline in either treatment arm. There were no side effects or adverse events. The authors concluded that supraphysiologic doses of melatonin do not positively affect tardive dyskinesia. However, considering that melatonin is a safe drug, it was felt that further studies are needed of higher doses and in patients with shorter disease duration before its use in the treatment of tardive dyskinesia is ruled out. Indeed, a year later [21] published the results of a second attempt to investigate the effects of melatonin treatment for tardive dyskinesia. Using a double-blind, placebo-controlled, crossover study, they evaluated the efficacy of 10 mg/d of melatonin for 6 weeks in 22 patients with both schizophrenia and significant tardive dyskinesia. The primary outcome measure was the change from baseline in AIMS score. Indeed, the decrease in AIMS score was 2.45 ± 1.92 for the melatonin and 0.77 ± 1.11 for the placebo treatment groups ($P<.001$). Treatment was safe and well tolerated by all patients. The authors observed then that this was the first clinical evidence for efficacy of melatonin in the treatment of tardive dyskinesia.

Carta et al [24] reviewed all available data on the treatment of tardive dyskinesia. They used a computer-generated search of the biomedical literature up to and including December 2002. Some evidence supports switching from typical neuroleptics to second generation antipsychotics in patients with tardive dyskinesia (particularly clozapine and olanzapine). Other than the new antipsychotics amongst tentative efforts to treat tardive dyskinesia with GABAergic compounds or the new anticholinergics, melatonin seems to be clinically useful. The authors recommended that future research should be directed to confirm the efficacy of these new drugs and to offer other treatment opportunities for patients.

Sleep

Since the 1970's there have been only 13 studies that either directly or indirectly examined sleep parameters amongst schizophrenia patients and melatonin. Only two of these studies directly addressed the effects of melatonin as an aid to the sleep disturbances so frequently reported by patients suffering from schizophrenia [25, 26]. A recent case report [27] emphasized that the period of the rest-activity rhythm, light-dark cycle, and melatonin rhythm was longer than 24 h in a schizophrenia patient. These circadian abnormalities may reinforce the altered sleep patterns and the problems of cognitive function and social engagement associated with schizophrenic.

Relying on testing the first –night-effect (subjects tendency to sleep worse than normal during their first night of polysomnographic sleep evaluation) as a reflection of flexible adaptation Shamir and colleagues [26] first demonstrated that administration of melatonin to patients suffering from chronic schizophrenia positively affected the first-night-effect. The group than went on [25] to study whether the association of insomnia with low or abnormal melatonin rhythms in patients with schizophrenia may be partially due to diminished melatonin output and thus corrected by melatonin replacement.

In the aforementioned study [25] melatonin replacement improved all of the following sleep variables: rest-derived sleep, sleep efficiency, shortened sleep latency and sleep duration. The authors had concluded that after taking into consideration the study's limitations it may tentatively be suggested that melatonin improves sleep efficiency in patients with schizophrenia.

Cognitive Dysfunction

There are a number of factors suggesting a relationship between decline of melatonin function and the deficits of dementia [28]. A comprehensive meta-analysis carried out by the Cochrane has been published recently [29]. In brief, the lines of evidence associating melatonin and cognition are as follows: 1) decline of serum melatonin levels to an even greater extent than in normal aging, 2) the breakdown of normal circadian rhythmicity in patients with dementia, 3) correlation between typical areas of cerebral atrophy in certain dementias (e.g. temporal lobes in Alzheimer's disease, and those areas containing melatonin receptors, 4) the known involvement of oxidative and amyloid-mediated brain damage in the pathogenesis of dementia coupled with antioxidant and antiamyloidogenic properties of melatonin, 5) melatonin has been reported to have both vasoconstricting and vasorelaxing properties. Vasoconstriction could also, theoretically, compromise cerebral circulation in older people with atherosclerosis. However, another study suggests melatonin may diminish the risk of hypoperfusion-induced cerebral ischemia by shifting the lower limit of cerebral blood flow autoregulation to a lower pressure level, improving the cerebrovascular dilatatory reserve, and thus widening the security margin and 6) anti-convulsant and neuro-protective effects have been reported for melatonin [29].

The previous brief background justified the undertaking of a systematic review of evidence relating to the clinical efficacy and safety of melatonin in the treatment of manifestations of dementia or cognitive impairment by the Cochrane foundation. The authors concluded that there is insufficient evidence to support the use of melatonin for treatment of cognitive impairment. However, results may be strengthened by longitudinal studies that examine the influence of melatonin over an extended time span. In addition, they suggest that future studies should not incorporate a cross over design due to the potential residual effect following cross over. Single interventions should be tested so that the effects can be clearly attributed to one intervention.

Conclusion

Despite over 50 years of study, the involvement of melatonin in the pathophysiology and treatment of schizophrenia is far from elucidated. Only sparse data is available and most of the sources are either anecdotal or limited by small sample size. Several findings do suggest that melatonin's treatment potential has not been fully explored in this chronic disabling disease.

REFERENCES

[1] Werneke U, Turner T, Priebe S. Complementary medicines in psychiatry: review of effectiveness and safety. *Br. J. Psychiatry* 2006; 188: 109-21.

[2] Lerner AB, Case JD, Takahashi Y. Isolation of melatonin and 5-methoxyindole-3-acetic acid from bovine pineal glands. *J. Biol. Chem.* 1960; 235: 1992-7.

[3] Arendt J. Melatonin. Clin Endocrinol (Oxf) 1988; 29: 205-29.

[4] Hardeland R, Pandi-Perumal SR, Cardinali DP. Melatonin. *Int. J. Biochem. Cell Biol.* 2006; 38: 313-6.

[5] Snyder SH, Borjigin J, Sassone-Corsi P. Discovering light effects on the brain. *Am. J. Psychiatry* 2006; 163: 771.

[6] Mueser KT, McGurk SR. Schizophrenia. *Lancet* 2004; 363: 2063-72.

[7] Altschule MD. Some effects of aqueous extracts of acetone-dried beef-pineal substance in chronic schizophrenia. *N Engl. J. Med.* 1957; 257: 919-22.

[8] Sandyk R. Tardive dyskinesia and the pineal gland. *Int. J. Neurosci.* 1988; 43: 111-4.

[9] Sandyk R, Kay SR. Pineal melatonin in schizophrenia: a review and hypothesis. *Schizophr. Bull.* 1990; 16: 653-62.

[10] Sandyk R. The pineal gland and the mode of onset of schizophrenia. *Int. J. Neurosci.* 1992; 67: 9-17.

[11] Pacchierotti C, Iapichino S, Bossini L, Pieraccini F, Castrogiovanni P. Melatonin in psychiatric disorders: a review on the melatonin involvement in psychiatry. *Front Neuroendocrinol.* 2001; 22: 18-32.

[12] Klein DC, Rowe J. Pineal gland in organ culture. I. Inhibition by harmine of serotonin-14C oxidation, accompanied by stimulation of melatonin-14C production. *Mol. Pharmacol.* 1970; 6: 164-71.

[13] Lynch HJ. Increase in rat pineal melatonin content following L-DOPA administration. *Life Sci.* 1973; 12: 145-151.

[14] McMillin D. The Treatment of Schizophrenia. Virginia A.R.E. Press, 1991.

[15] Bersani G, Mameli M, Garavini A, Pancheri P, Nordio M. Reduction of night/day difference in melatonin blood levels as a possible disease-related index in schizophrenia. *Neuro. Endocrinol. Lett.* 2003; 24: 181-4.

[16] Vigano D, Lissoni P, Rovelli F, Roselli MG, Malugani F, Gavazzeni C, Conti A, Maestroni G. A study of light/dark rhythm of melatonin in relation to cortisol and prolactin secretion in schizophrenia. *Neuro. Endocrinol. Lett.* 2001; 22: 137-41.

[17] Rao ML, Gross G, Strebel B, Halaris A, Huber G, Braunig P, Marler M. Circadian rhythm of tryptophan, serotonin, melatonin, and pituitary hormones in schizophrenia. *Biol. Psychiatry* 1994; 35: 151-63.

[18] Schwartz PJ, Erk SD. Regulation of central dopamine-2 receptor sensitivity by a proportional control thermostat in humans. *Psychiatry Res.* 2004; 127: 19-26.

[19] Schneider-Mayerson A. Shedding light on suicide and schizophrenia: hormonal changes and vitamin deficiencies are implicated. *Psychology Today* 2002.

[20] Lohr JB, Kuczenski R, Niculescu AB. Oxidative mechanisms and tardive dyskinesia. *CNS Drugs* 2003; 17: 47-62.

[21] Shamir E, Barak Y, Shalman I, Laudon M, Zisapel N, Tarrasch R, Elizur A, Weizman R. Melatonin treatment for tardive dyskinesia: a double-blind, placebo-controlled, crossover study. *Arch Gen. Psychiatry* 2001; 58: 1049-52.

[22] Zhang XY, Zhou DF, Cao LY, Xu CQ, Chen DC, Wu GY. The effect of vitamin E treatment on tardive dyskinesia and blood superoxide dismutase: a double-blind placebo-controlled trial. *J. Clin. Psychopharmacol.* 2004; 24: 83-6.

[23] Shamir E, Barak Y, Plopsky I, Zisapel N, Elizur A, Weizman A. Is melatonin treatment effective for tardive dyskinesia? *J. Clin. Psychiatry* 2000; 61: 556-8.

[24] Carta MG, Hardoy MC, Dell'Osso L, Carpiniello B. [Tardive dyskinesia: review of the literature]. *Clin. Ter.* 2004; 155: 127-33.

[25] Shamir E, Laudon M, Barak Y, Anis Y, Rotenberg V, Elizur A, Zisapel N. Melatonin improves sleep quality of patients with chronic schizophrenia. *J. Clin. Psychiatry* 2000; 61: 373-7.

[26] Shamir E, Rotenberg VS, Laudon M, Zisapel N, Elizur A. First-night effect of melatonin treatment in patients with chronic schizophrenia. *J. Clin. Psychopharmacol.* 2000; 20: 691-4.

[27] Wulff K, Joyce E, Middleton B, Dijk DJ, Foster RG. The suitability of actigraphy, diary data, and urinary melatonin profiles for quantitative assessment of sleep disturbances in schizophrenia: a case report. *Chronobiol. Int.* 2006; 23: 485-95.

[28] Canadian study of health and aging: study methods and prevalence of dementia. *Cmaj* 1994; 150: 899-913.

[29] Jansen SL, Forbes DA, Duncan V, Morgan DG. Melatonin for cognitive impairment. *Cochrane Database Syst. Rev.* 2006: CD003802.

INDEX

B

C

D

G

H

I

J

K

L

M

N

O

P

S

T

U